STOP PLAYIN', GO VEGAN

GETTING SERIOUS WITH HEALTHY VEGAN RECIPES TO PREVENT AND REVERSE DISEASE!

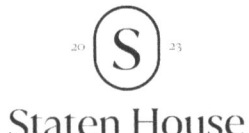

Staten House

ISBN 979-8-89686-581-0 (pbk.) -- 979-8-89686-583-4 (epub)
Published by Staten House

1-Cooking-Health-Nutrition

Cover Photography: Gabriel Trofort
Food Photography: Gene Setzer, Ruby Lathon

www.StopPlayinGoVegan.com

The information in Stop Playin', Go Vegan: Getting Serious with Healthy Vegan Recipes to Prevent and Reverse Disease! is intended for educational and informational purposes only. The recipes, nutritional insights, and health-related discussions are based on the author's personal experience and research. This book is not intended to diagnose, treat, cure, or prevent any disease.

The author is not a medical doctor, and the content provided should not be considered a substitute for professional medical advice, diagnosis, or treatment. Always consult with a qualified healthcare provider before making any dietary or lifestyle changes, especially if you are pregnant or on medication. The author and publisher disclaim any liability for any adverse effects resulting directly or indirectly from the use of the information in this book. Every individual is unique, and results may vary.

STOP PLAYIN', GO VEGAN

GETTING SERIOUS WITH HEALTHY VEGAN RECIPES TO PREVENT AND REVERSE DISEASE!

RUBY LATHON, PHD

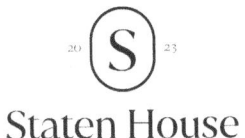

Staten House

DEDICATION

To my mom (Henrietta Lathon), who taught me how to cook from the soul and showed me that food is more than just nourishment, it's love, tradition, and the glue that brings families together. Your wisdom and warmth continue to inspire every meal I make.

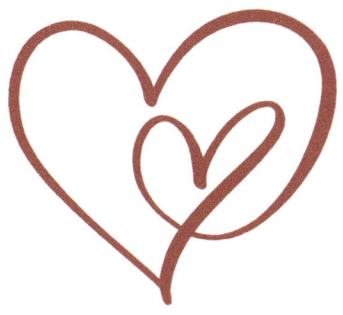

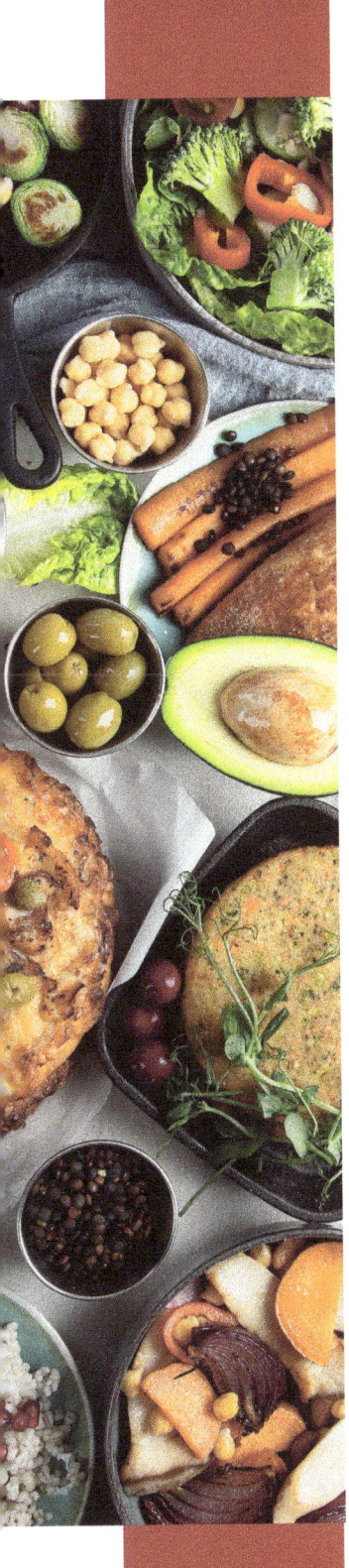

Stop Playin', Go Vegan:
Getting Serious with Healthy Vegan Recipes to Prevent and
Reverse Disease!

The table of

CONTENTS

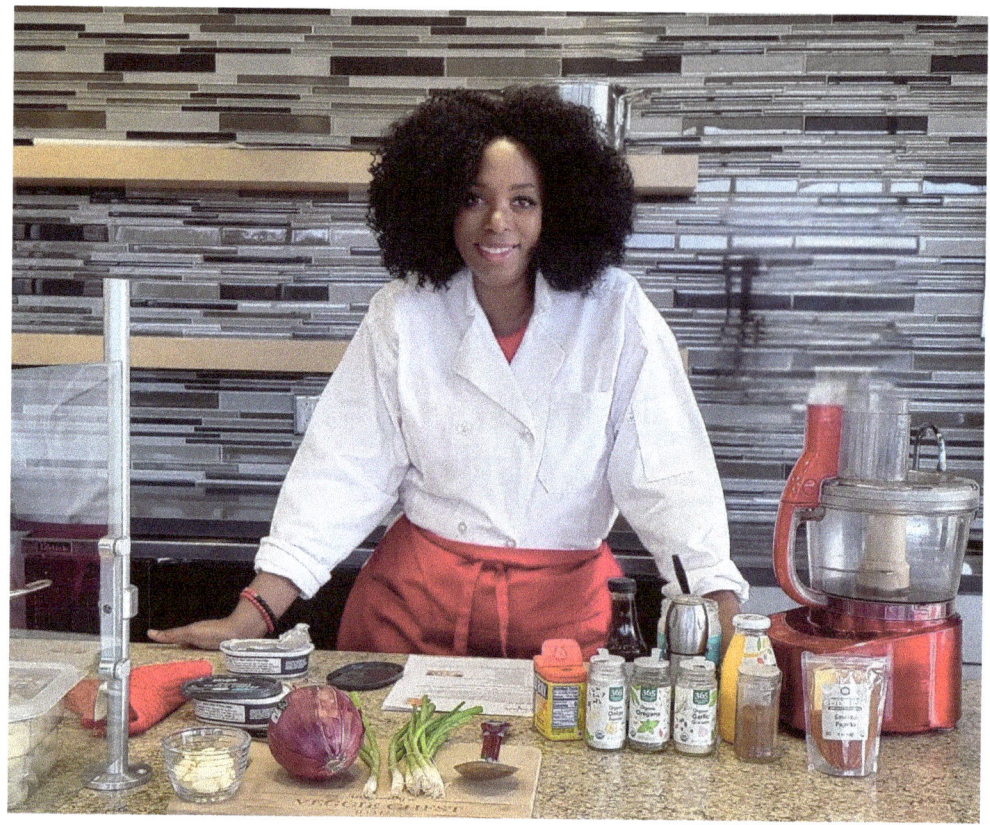

1. INTRODUCTION

When I first transitioned to a plant-based lifestyle, I had no idea how powerful food could be. I was searching for a way to heal. After being diagnosed with thyroid cancer, I dove deep into the world of nutrition, determined to take control of my health. What I discovered changed everything.

Food is medicine. The right foods can nourish, restore, and certainly help the body heal. Through my own journey, I developed and perfected recipes that are not only loaded with nutrients but also full of bold flavors and comforting familiarity. Stop Playin', Go Vegan is a collection of over 110 of those recipes, dishes designed to support your health while making every meal something to look forward to.

This book is more than just a cookbook. It's a guide to using plant-based foods to help prevent and even reverse some chronic illnesses. Whether you're here to improve your health, boost your energy, or simply enjoy delicious, wholesome meals, you'll find everything you need, immune-boosting meals, cancer-fighting dishes, gut-friendly probiotic-rich recipes, thyroid-supporting foods, and even indulgent treats for when you want to satisfy a craving.

If you've been thinking about going plant-based but don't know where to start, I've got you. If you're already vegan but want to take your health to the next level, you're in the right place. No matter where you are on your journey, this book will help you make plant-based eating easy, enjoyable, and most importantly, deeply nourishing.

So let's get serious about feeling good, living well, and loving what's on our plates. It's time to Stop Playin' and Go Vegan!

With Love,

Dr. Ruby

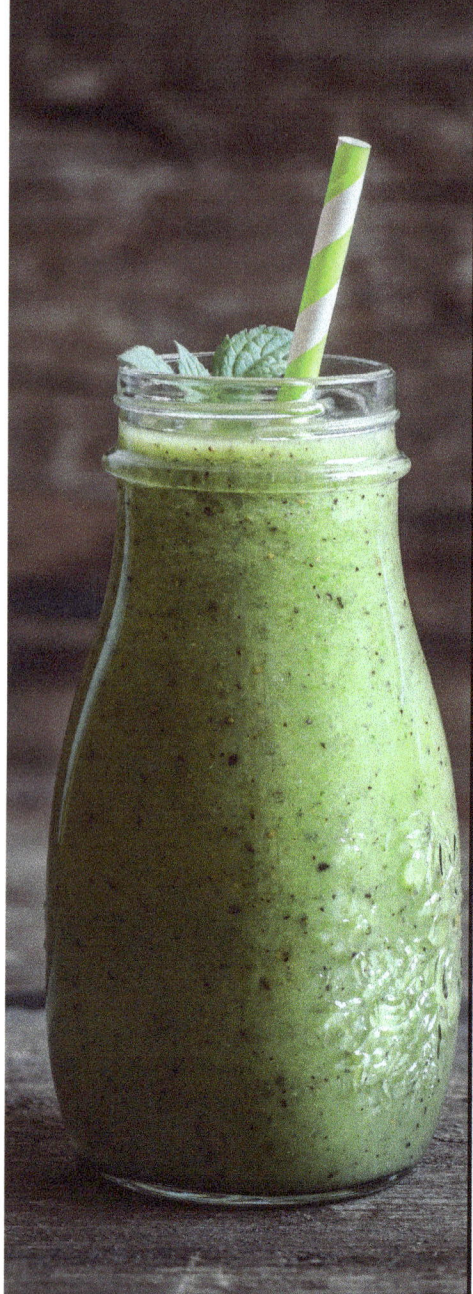

*Nourish your body,
sip by sip.*

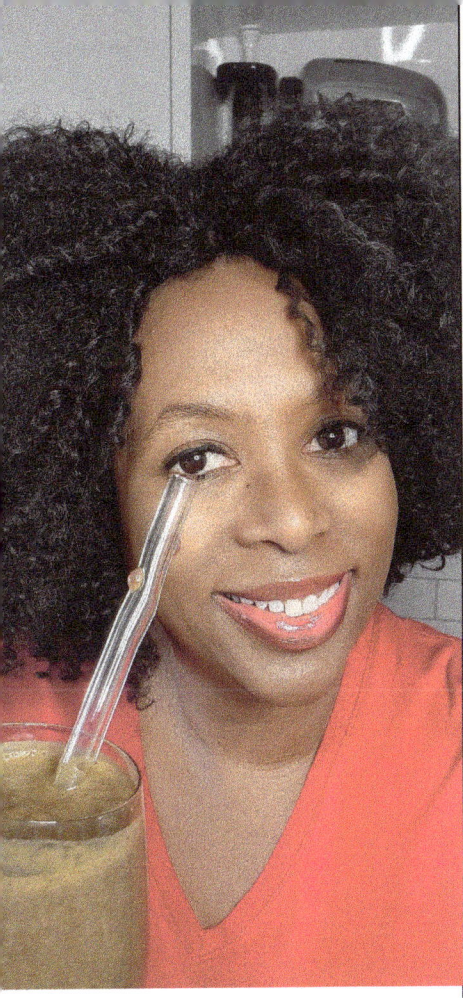

THE BASICS

Smoothies are not just for breakfast! I enjoy these nutrient-dense delights for lunch, dinner, and even as snacks. They're a treasure trove of health benefits. Quick to whip up, loaded with nutrients, and absolutely delicious, these recipes will help you fend off illness and embrace a lively lifestyle.

You might be curious about **the difference between juicing and blending**. The scoop: juicing extracts the liquid and discards the fiber, providing a concentrated nutrient boost. Blending retains all that beneficial fiber, which is fantastic for digestion and helps you feel satisfied. Both methods have their benefits in a balanced diet, so I've included some juicing recipes as well. They're ideal for when you want a quick nutrient surge without the extra bulk.

After years of exploring how plant-based nutrition can enhance health, I can assure you that what you drink is just as crucial as what you eat. These smoothies are not only delicious; they're powerful potions against inflammation, chronic diseases, and fatigue.

Time saver: don't hesitate to double the smoothie recipes. Smoothies and juices store wonderfully in the fridge for 24-48 hours, allowing you to prepare ahead and have a nutritious meal or snack ready when you need it. Prepped, done.

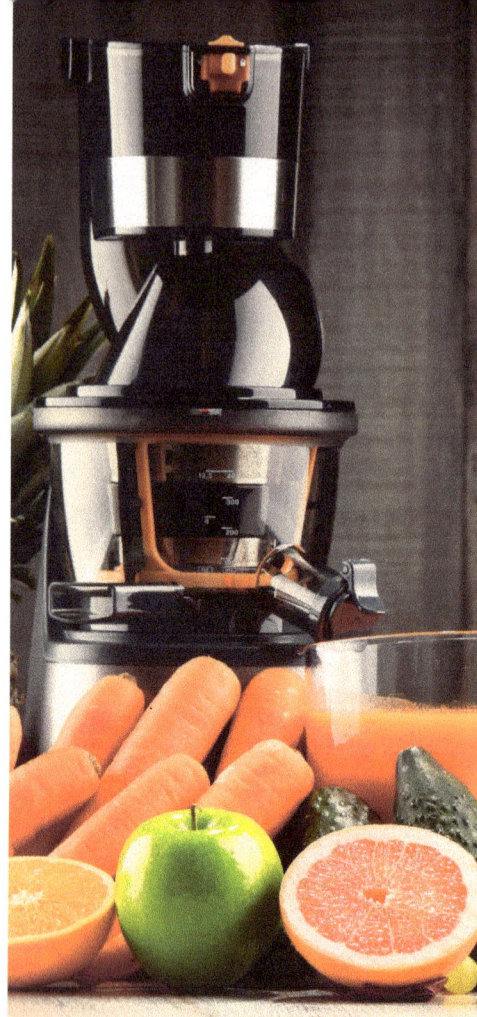

Key Benefits of Smoothies: Your Blended Health Companion

1. Nutrient Release: Blending breaks down plant structures, allowing your body to absorb all those fantastic nutrients.
2. Hydration Champion: Smoothies are not only delicious but also combine the benefits of water and a natural multivitamin in one refreshing drink.
3. Digestive-Friendly Fiber: Each sip supports your gut health and keeps you feeling full for longer periods. Their full of prebiotic fiber that helps balance your gut bacteria.
4. Disease-Defending Properties: High in antioxidants, they protect the cells, and fight inflammation and oxidative stress.

Key Benefits of Juicing: Your Liquid Wellness Weapon

1. Nutritional Powerhouse: Imagine squeezing an entire farmer's market into a single glass - that's the magic of juicing.
2. Digestive Break: By removing fiber, juices require minimal digestive effort, making them ideal for those recovering from illness or who have sensitive digestive systems.
3. Quick Nutrition Boost: Without fiber, the body can quickly absorb the nutrients, providing a quick dose of potent nutrients and a fast energy boost.
4. Detoxification Support: The concentrated nutrients in juices can help support the body in eliminating toxins.

Buuuuut, what about the sugar?

So, you're worried about all the fruit sugar, right? When it comes to smoothies, we're not just tossing in a bunch of fruit and calling it a day. We're creating balanced, nutritional power food. So, let's break this down:

1. **Fiber is your friend:** Unlike juice, smoothies keep all that good fiber intact. Fiber slows down sugar absorption, so you're not getting a crazy blood sugar spike.
2. **Greens are the real MVPs:** Adding leafy greens like collards or kale to your smoothie help balance out the fruit sugars. For an added bonus, add a green powder that includes ingredients like spirulina, chlorella and moringa.
3. **High protein plant foods seal the deal:** Protein further slows down sugar absorption and keeps you feeling full. Adding in some chia seeds, hemp hearts, flax seeds, pumpkin seeds or an organic plant-based protein powder will not only up the protein and nutrients, it keeps the smoothie from becoming a sugar bomb.
4. **Whole fruit ≠ added sugar:** Whole fruit contains natural sugars balanced by fiber and nutrients, metabolized differently than isolated sugars.

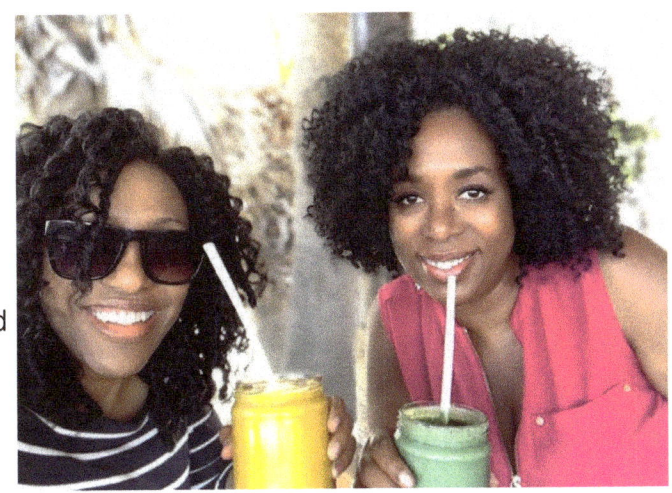

Sis and me—getting our smoothie fix even on vacay.

Now, for juicing, we play it a little differently:
1. **Veggie-forward:** We're talking mostly low-glycemic vegetables. Think cucumber, celery, cabbage, kale.
2. **Fruit and sweet veggies as supporting actors:** A bit of apple, pear or beets? Yes, but just enough to make it tasty without going overboard and making it too sweet..
3. **Strategic choices:** When you use fruit, opt for lower-sugar options like green apples, pears, lemons, or limes.

If you have specific health concerns or conditions, these guideline may change a bit. Always talk with your healthcare provider. But for most people, a well-crafted smoothie or juice can be a fantastic addition to a healthy diet.

Blueberry Banana Smoothie

This smoothie is so delicious; it tastes more like a milk shake!

INGREDIENTS

1/2 cup   organic blueberries
1   banana
1/2 cup   pumpkin seed milk
1 tbsp   hemp seeds
1/2 cup   ice

DIRECTIONS

1. Place all the ingredients in a blender.
2. Blend on high speed until smooth.

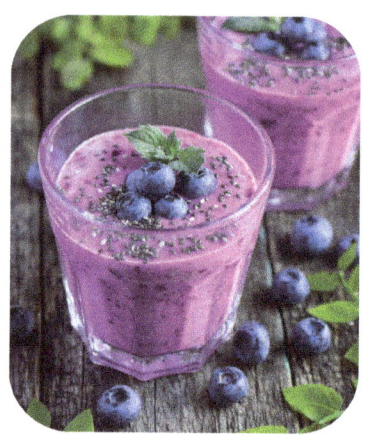

Blueberries' anthocyanins may enhance memory, while hemp seeds' omega-3s support focus—making this a perfect morning or post-workout recharge.

Pumpkin Seed Milk

½ cup pumpkin seeds
½ cup pitted dates
½ tsp vanilla extract or half vanilla bean
3-4 cups water

Directions: Place pumpkin seeds, dates, vanilla, and water in blender and blend until smooth. Milk will keep for 5 days, refrigerated.

SERVINGS	TIME	LEVEL	KCAL	FIBER	CARB	FAT	PROTEIN
2	10 mins	easy	4	7g	39g	3g	3g

Cleansing Citrus Smoothie

I love this vibrant, detoxifying blend that supports digestion and immunity. The cayenne give this a nice kick!

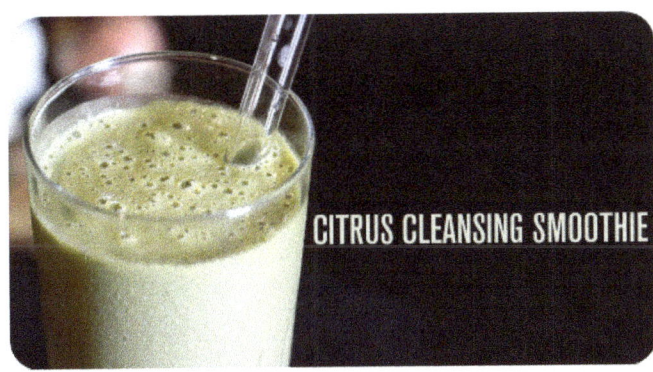

CITRUS CLEANSING SMOOTHIE

Cayenne's capsaicin triggers a gentle metabolic spark and may support immunity by promoting healthy inflammation response.

INGREDIENTS

1	ripe mango, peeled, cut into chunks
1	orange
1	lemon
1	banana (optional)
2-3	kale leaves
1/2 inch	ginger
2-3 tbsp	hemp seeds
1/2 cup	ice
3/4 cup	water or coconut water
1/8 tsp	cayenne pepper

DIRECTIONS

1. Add all ingredients to a blender, starting with leafy greens.
2. Blend until smooth.
3. Serve immediately.

SERVINGS	TIME	LEVEL	KCAL	FIBER	CARB	FAT	PROTEIN
2	10 mins	easy	303	11g	56g	9g	8g

Cinnamon Spice Apple Smoothie

This smoothie is loaded with immune allies: vitamin C from lemon and apples, antiviral cinnamon and cloves, and zinc-rich hemp seeds for white blood cell support

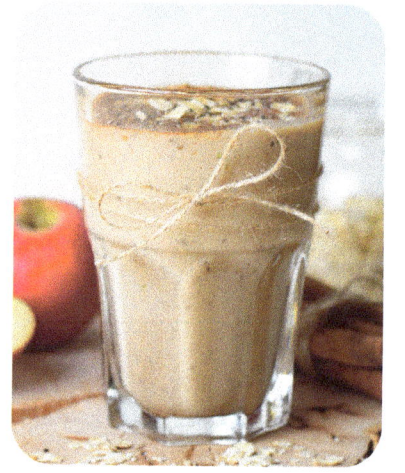

Moringa's iron helps oxygenate infection-fighting cells.

INGREDIENTS

1	golden apple, unpeeled & seeded
1	banana, peeled
1/2	lemon, juiced
2-4	dates
1/2 tsp	cinnamon
1/4 tsp	coriander
Dash	cloves
2 tbsp	hempseeds
1	Brazil nut
1/2 tsp	moringa powder
1 handful	organic lettuce greens
3/4 cup	water or coconut water
1/2 cup	ice

DIRECTIONS

1. Add all ingredients to a blender, starting with leafy greens.
2. Blend until smooth.
3. Serve immediately or store in glass jar and refrigerate.

SERVINGS	TIME	LEVEL	KCAL	FIBER	CARB	FAT	PROTEIN
2	10 mins	easy	197	9g	67g	11g	7g

Simple Green Smoothie

A no-fuss, nutrient-dense blend that's as easy to make as it is to love.

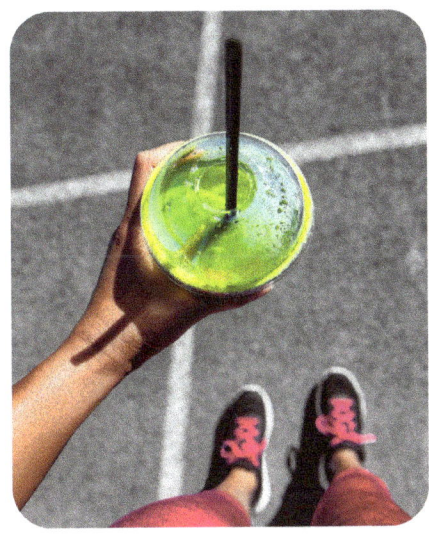

Kiwi skin adds extra fiber, ginger soothes digestion, and hemp seeds provide a complete protein, all in one refreshing blend.

INGREDIENTS

1	kiwi, washed and unpeeled
1	clementine, peeled
1	banana, peeled
1 inch	fresh ginger
2	kale leaves with stems
3 tbsp	hemp seeds
1 cup	water or coconut water
1/2 cup	ice

DIRECTIONS

1. Add all ingredients to a blender, starting with kale.
2. Blend until smooth.
3. Serve immediately or store in glass jar with lid and refrigerate.

SERVINGS	TIME	LEVEL	KCAL	FIBER	CARB	FAT	PROTEIN
2	10 mins	easy	197	5g	28g	8g	7g

Pineapple Coconut Smoothie

Tropical, creamy, and sneaking in greens without a trace.
(Even collard-haters won't know.)

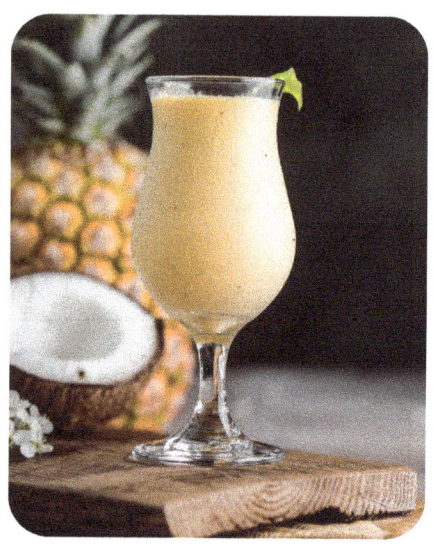

INGREDIENTS

1 cup	fresh or frozen pineapple, peeled
1	orange, peeled
1	banana, peeled
1 inch	fresh ginger
1	large collard green leaf
1/4 cup	fresh coconut meat or 3 tbsp unsweetened, dried shredded coconut
2 tbsp	pumpkin seeds
3/4 cup	coconut water
1/2 cup	ice

DIRECTIONS

1. Add all ingredients to a blender, starting with collard greens.
2. Blend until smooth.
3. Serve immediately or store in glass jar and refrigerate.

Pineapple's bromelain aids digestion, coconut meat adds healthy fats, and pumpkin seeds boost zinc for immunity—all while tasting like vacation.

SERVINGS	TIME	LEVEL	KCAL	FIBER	CARB	FAT	PROTEIN
2	10 mins	easy	197	5g	28g	8g	7g

Chocolate Cherry Smoothie

Raw cacao packs more antioxidants than blueberries, and its magnesium helps ease stress, and cherries' melatonin makes this a relaxation dream team.

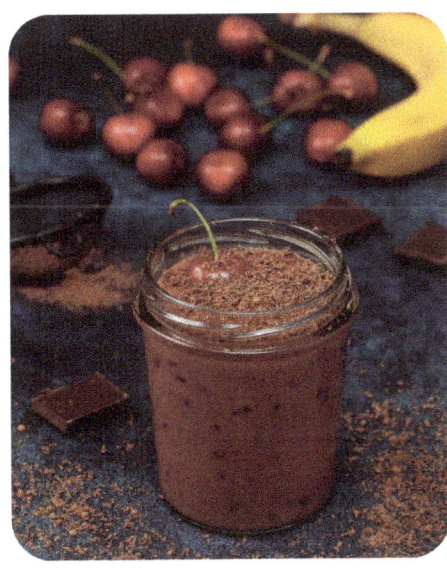

Frozen cherries thicken the blend while keeping it icy-cold, like a milkshake but better.

INGREDIENTS

1.5 cups	frozen dark sweet cherries
2	bananas (fresh or frozen)
2 tbsp	raw cacao powder
1/2 cup	baby spinach, packed
1/2 cup	coconut water or coconut milk
1/2 cup	ice

DIRECTIONS

1. Add all ingredients to a blender, starting with the baby spinach.
2. Blend until smooth.
3. Serve immediately or store in glass jar and refrigerate.

SERVINGS	TIME	LEVEL	KCAL	FIBER	CARB	FAT	PROTEIN
2	10 mins	easy	197	7g	49g	7g	4g

Muscle Building Smoothie

A post-workout (or anytime) blend that fuels recovery with plant-based protein, healthy fats, and inflammation-soothing ingredients.

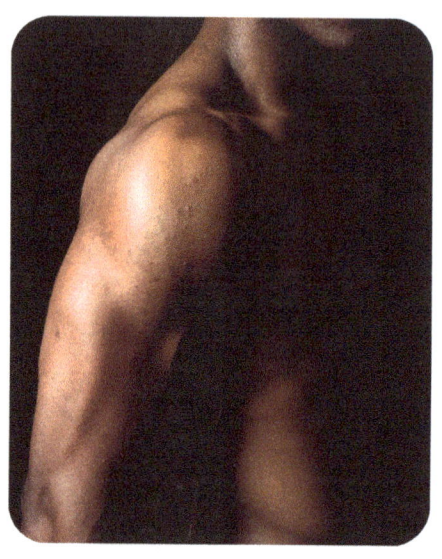

INGREDIENTS

1 cup	organic frozen berry mix
1	banana
2	kale leaves or handful mixed greens
3 tbsp	hemp seeds
3 tbsp	pumpkin seeds
1 tsp	moringa powder
1/4 cup	coconut meat
1/4 cup	almonds (optional)
2	dates, pitted
1 inch	ginger
1 cup	water or coconut water

DIRECTIONS

1. Add all ingredients to a blender, starting with leafy greens.
2. Blend until smooth.
3. Serve immediately or store in glass jar and refrigerate.

Hemp and pumpkin seeds deliver complete protein + zinc for repair, moringa adds iron for oxygen flow, and ginger cools post-workout inflammation—no powders needed.

SERVINGS	TIME	LEVEL	KCAL	FIBER	CARB	FAT	PROTEIN
2	10 mins	easy	378	9g	50g	18g	14g

Pumpkin Seed Protein Smoothie

A whole-food protein boost, with pumpkin seeds, moringa, and real fruit (no synthetic powders).

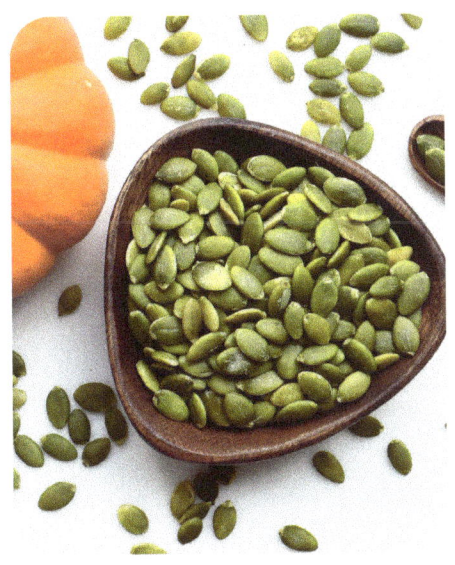

Pumpkin seeds are a complete plant protein—just 2 tablespoons give you 5g protein, plus magnesium for muscles and zinc for immunity.

INGREDIENTS

1 cup	frozen organic berries or ½ cup cherries
2	bananas
2 tbsp	raw pumpkin seed powder
1 tsp	moringa powder
1/4 cup	walnuts
1	date, pitted
1 cup	water or coconut water

DIRECTIONS

1. Add all ingredients to a blender, starting with bananas.
2. Blend until smooth.
3. Serve immediately or store in glass jar and refrigerate.

SERVINGS	TIME	LEVEL	KCAL	FIBER	CARB	FAT	PROTEIN
2	10 mins	easy	454	10g	55g	24g	14g

Refreshing Grapefruit Recovery Smoothie

Grapefruit has a low glycemic index (GI 25), so its natural sugars are absorbed slowly, helping balance blood sugar while delivering a vitamin C punch.

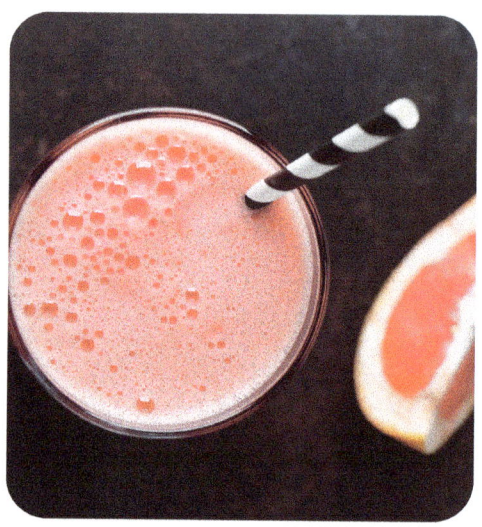

Half a grapefruit delivers 64% of your daily vitamin C, with a metabolism-boosting bonus from naringenin, a flavonoid that supports fat burning.

INGREDIENTS

1-2	Ruby Red grapefruits, peeled and quartered
3 tbsp	pumpkin seeds
1	date, pitted
1/4 cup	ice

DIRECTIONS

1. Add all ingredients to a blender, starting with the grapefruit.
2. Blend until smooth.
3. Serve immediately.

SERVINGS	TIME	LEVEL	KCAL	FIBER	CARB	FAT	PROTEIN
2	10 mins	easy	216	7g	37g	7g	6g

Prickly Pear Pineapple Cooler

This isn't just a poolside drink, it's a hydration hack with skin-glowing and gut-loving perks!

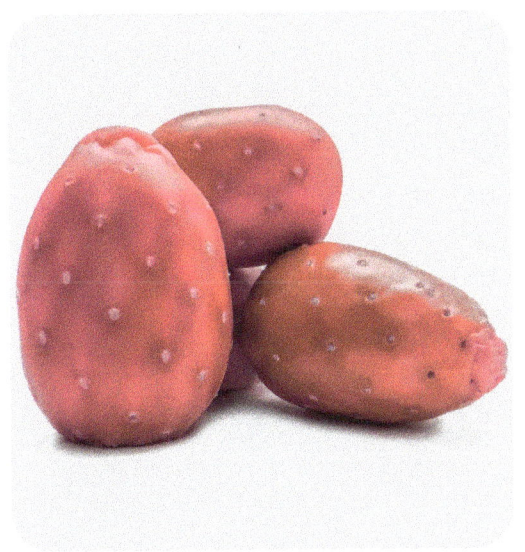

INGREDIENTS

1	prickly pear, peeled
1 cup	chopped pineapple, peeled
1/2 cup	baby spinach
3 tbsp	hemp seeds
1/4 cup	coconut water
1/2 cup	ice
3-4	fresh mint leaves for garnish

Prickly pear's betalains fight inflammation, pineapple's bromelain aids digestion, and hemp seeds add omega-3s for cellular repair—hydration with a purpose.

DIRECTIONS

1. Add all ingredients to a blender, starting with the baby spinach.
2. Blend until smooth.
3. Serve immediately.

SERVINGS	TIME	LEVEL	KCAL	FIBER	CARB	FAT	PROTEIN
2	10 mins	easy	196	5g	22g	8g	6g

Watermelon Lemon Splash

My favorite summer cleansing drink. It's such an easy cleanse.

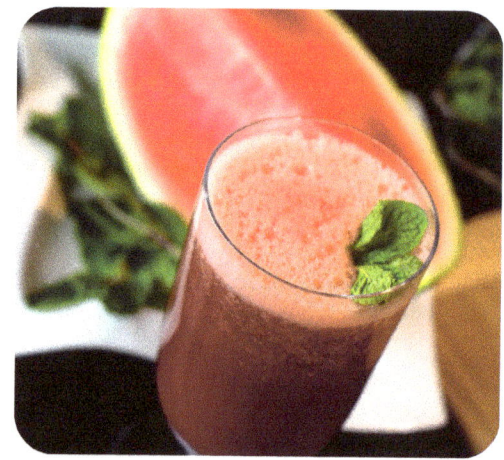

Why I Love It:
Watermelon's citrulline supports
blood flow, while lemon's D-
limonene helps liver detox. Each sip
brings a lighter, brighter feeling.

INGREDIENTS

1/2	medium watermelon, peeled
2	lemons, peeled and cut in half
1 cup	fresh mint leaves
2 tbsp	raw agave nectar (optional: omit when cleansing; include when enjoying or if you prefer more sweetness)

DIRECTIONS

1. Add all ingredients to a blender.
2. Blend until smooth.
3. Serve immediately or store in refrigerator.

SERVINGS	TIME	LEVEL	KCAL	FIBER	CARB	FAT	PROTEIN
6-8	15 mins	easy	62	1g	16g	0g	1g

Anti-Inflammatory Parsley Ginger Juice

One of my go-to easy detox juices that cleanses blood, fights inflammation, and floods my body with antioxidants.

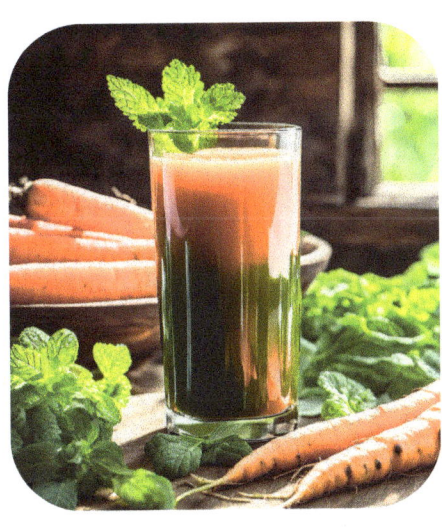

INGREDIENTS

6-8	organic carrots, washed and unpeeled
1 bunch	parsley, washed
3 inches	fresh ginger

Parsley acts as a natural blood cleanser, aiding in heavy metal detox, while ginger's potent anti-inflammatory compounds (like gingerols) soothe digestion and oxidative stress.

DIRECTIONS

1. Place the ingredients in the juicer, starting with the ginger, then the parsley, and finishing with the carrots.
2. Serve immediately, or store in a glass jar in the coldest part of your refrigerator.

SERVINGS	TIME	LEVEL	KCAL	FIBER	CARB	FAT	PROTEIN
2	10 mins	easy	96	2g	24g	0g	2g

Restore Cabbage Apple Juice

My favorite cancer fighting elixir, a science-backed trio (cabbage, apple, ginger) filled with compounds that may help starve and shield cells from damage.

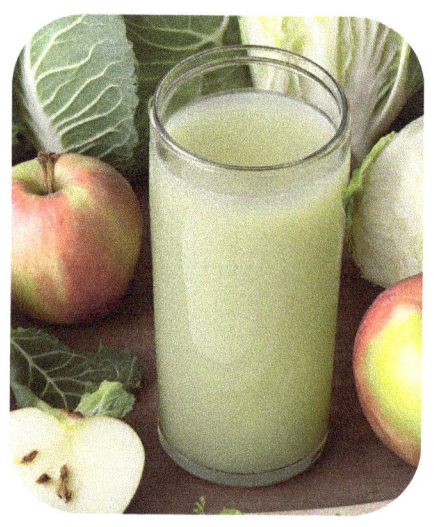

INGREDIENTS

1	small cabbage or ½ large cabbage
6	organic apples, unpeeled
3 inches	fresh ginger root

Cabbage's sulforaphane, apple's quercetin, and ginger's 6-ginerol synergize to combat oxidative stress, reduce inflammation, and support detox pathways—key mechanisms in cancer prevention.

DIRECTIONS

1. Place items in a juicer, starting with the ginger, then the cabbage and finishing with the apples.
2. Serve immediately, or store in a glass jar in the coldest part of your refrigerator.

SERVINGS	TIME	LEVEL	KCAL	FIBER	CARB	FAT	PROTEIN
2-4	15 mins	easy	96	2g	24g	0g	2g

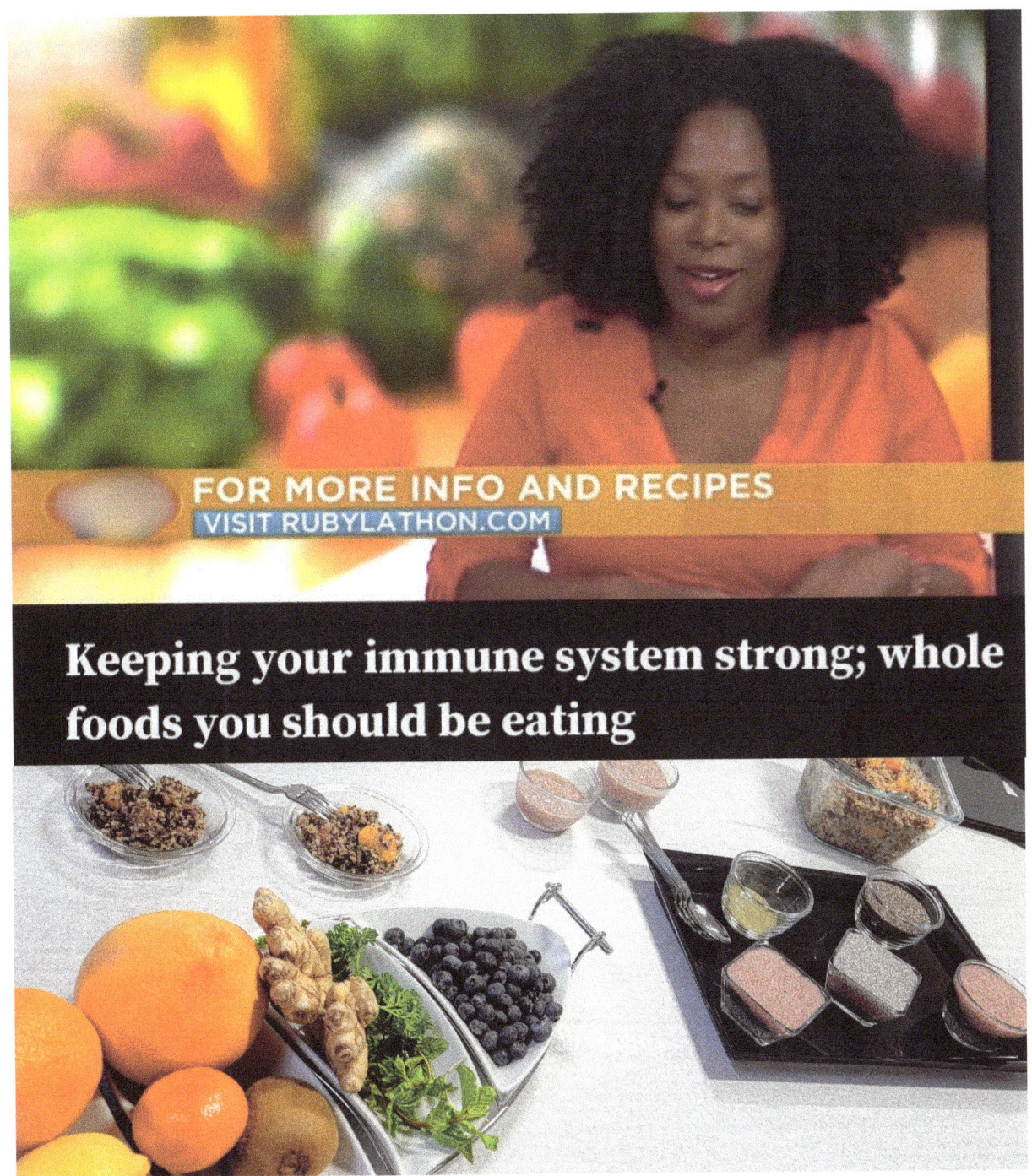

FOR MORE INFO AND RECIPES
VISIT RUBYLATHON.COM

Keeping your immune system strong; whole foods you should be eating

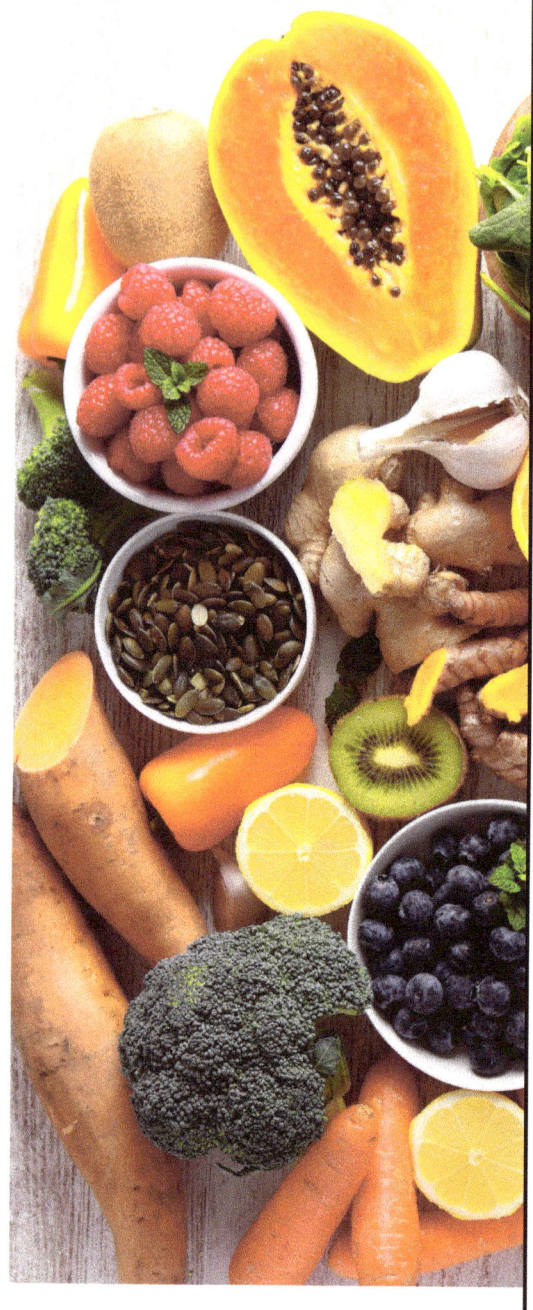

Let food be your shield.

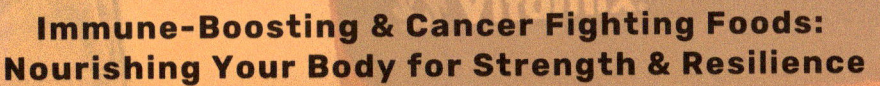

Immune-Boosting & Cancer Fighting Foods:
Nourishing Your Body for Strength & Resilience

Our immune system is our body's first line of defense, working tirelessly to protect us from illness and disease. The good news? We have the power to strengthen and support it through the food we eat. In this chapter, we'll focus on the incredible, plant-based foods that provide the essential vitamins, minerals, and antioxidants needed to fortify your immune system. From vitamin C-packed citrus to immune-boosting herbs and spices, these recipes are designed to help your body stay strong, resilient, and ready to fight off anything that comes its way.

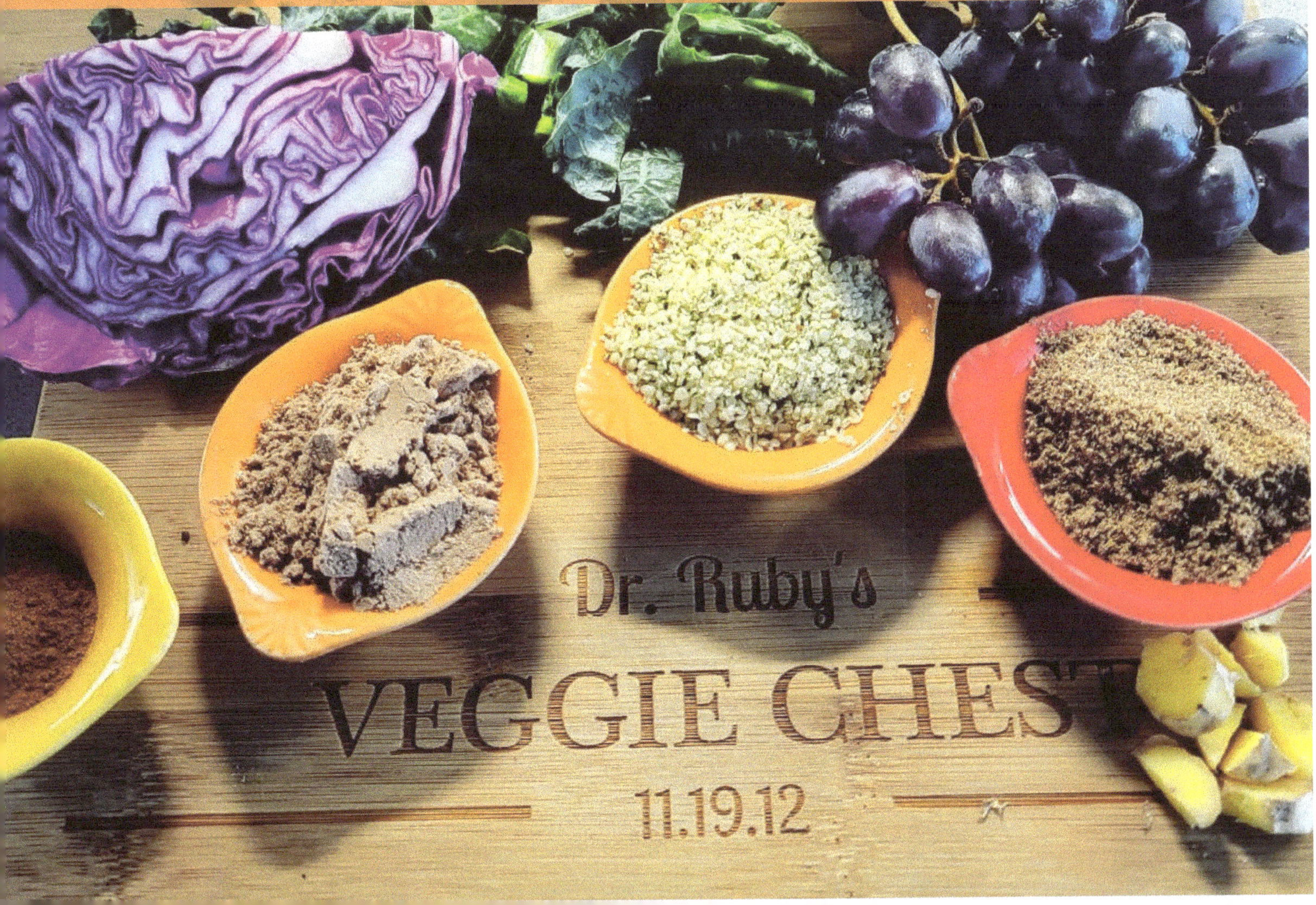

Dr. Ruby's
VEGGIE CHEST
11.19.12

Shredded Beet Jicama Salad with Lime Dressing

Not a fan of raw beets? This salad might change your mind. Crispy jicama and a splash of lime make a zesty combo—with bonus heart-healthy benefits

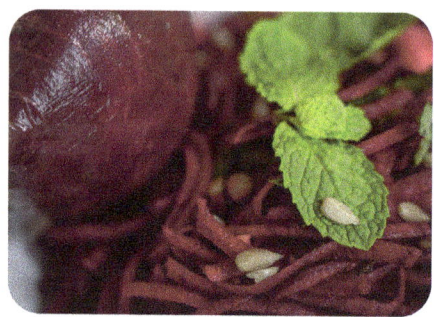

Beets are rich in nitrates, which support heart health and improve circulation.

INGREDIENTS

3 med	beets, peeled, shredded (medium to fine shreds, smaller is better
1 med	jicama, peeled and julienned into 1/2 inch strips
2 tsp	raw agave nectar
1 tsp	brown rice vinegar
1/2 tsp	cayenne pepper
2	limes, juiced
1/4 cup	mint leaves (cut in 1/4 inch ribbons)
1/4 cup	raw sunflower seeds

DIRECTIONS

1. Peel beets and then shred with a grater or food processor; Peel and slice jicama.
2. To prepare the dressing: Mix lime juice, rice vinegar, agave nectar, mint leaves and cayenne in a bowl, whisk well.
3. Pour over beets and jicama; mix until well coated.
4. Top with sunflower seeds.

SERVINGS	TIME	LEVEL	KCAL	FIBER	CARB	FAT	PROTEIN
3	25 mins	Medium	236	17g	41g	7g	7g

Broccoli Cranberry Medley with Poppy Seed Dressing

This is one of my favorite super easy salads! It's so nourishing, refreshing and crunchy!

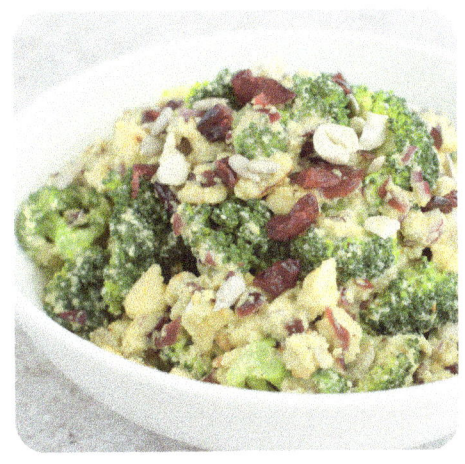

These flavorful alliums deliver a double punch: antioxidants to calm inflammation and organosulfur compounds for detox support.

INGREDIENTS

1 head	broccoli, washed, cut into florets
3	medium shallots, thinly sliced
1/2 cup	dried cranberries
3/4 cup	Creamy Poppy Seed Dressing (recipe on page 95)
1/2 cup	sunflower or pumpkin seeds
1/2 tsp	sea salt or to taste

DIRECTIONS

1. Put broccoli florets and stems into a food processor and pulse 2 to 3 times until broccoli is in small pieces, but not mushy. Alternatively, cut broccoli into small pieces with a knife.
2. Mix in shallots, cranberries and dressing until well coated.
3. Add sea salt to taste.
4. Serve immediately or store in refrigerator,

SERVINGS	TIME	LEVEL	KCAL	FIBER	CARB	FAT	PROTEIN
3	20 mins	easy	291	10g	49g	9g	11g

Cucumber Parsley Salad

You've probably noticed by now, raw, crunchy, and refreshing is my kind of theme. This cucumber parsley salad might seem unconventional, but it's so good.

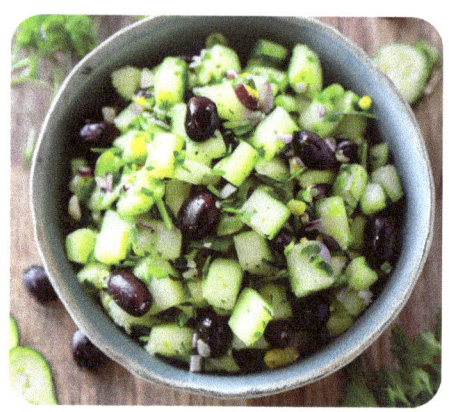

Parsley is a natural blood cleanser, rich in antioxidants and chlorophyll, which help detoxify the body.

INGREDIENTS

1	cucumber, diced
1 cup	parsley, chopped
2	green onions, chopped
1/2 cup	Kalamata olives, sliced
1/2 tsp	sea salt or to taste
3 tbsp	red wine vinegar
1 tbsp	lemon juice
3 tbsp	plain or garlic hummus, prepared

Optional: Add 1/2 cup of garbanzo beans or 3-bean mix (garbanzos, kidney beans and cannellini beans)

DIRECTIONS

1. Place all ingredients, except hummus in bowl and mix until well incorporated.
2. Top with hummus. Serve cold or at room temperature.

SERVINGS	TIME	LEVEL	KCAL	FIBER	CARB	FAT	PROTEIN
3	20 mins	easy	64	2g	7g	3g	3g

Forbidden Sesame Rice Pilaf

Black rice earned the name "Forbidden Rice" because, in ancient China, it was reserved exclusively for the emperor & nobility; commoners were forbidden from eating it. Its elite status came from scarcity, nutrition, and links to long life.

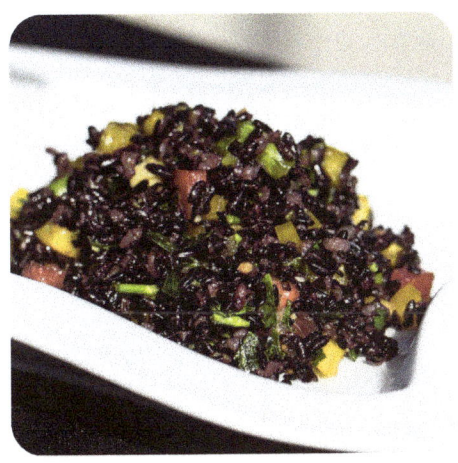

Black rice contains more protein than most other rice varieties, with about 9 grams per cooked cup.

INGREDIENTS

1.5 cup	organic black rice
1 med	tomatoes, diced
3	green onions, chopped
1/4 cup	cilantro, chopped
1 clove	garlic, minced
1/2	yellow bell pepper, diced
1	ripe avocado, diced
2 tbsp	lemon juice
1/4 tsp	sea salt
1 tsp	black or white sesame seeds

DIRECTIONS

1. Soak rice overnight or 8 hours. Drain and rinse. Start with very warm water.
2. Add rice and all other ingredients to a bowl and gently stir until all ingredients are well mixed.
3. Serve chilled or room temperature as a side item or main dish.

SERVINGS	TIME	LEVEL	KCAL	FIBER	CARB	FAT	PROTEIN
4	20 mins	easy	350	6g	62g	9g	9g

Collard Green & Black Rice Tacos

Never thought I'd eat raw collards—now I'm hooked! These leafy wraps replace flour tortillas with zero guilt, plus a mega fiber and nutrient boost.

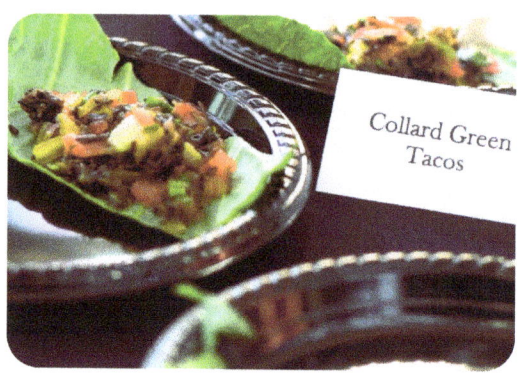

Collard Green Tacos

Rich in vitamin C and sulforaphane (a cancer-fighting compound), raw collards provide cellular defense.

INGREDIENTS

8 med	collard greens, stems removed
1 cup	broccoli or radish sprouts
1.5 cups	black rice (aka Forbidden rice)
1 med	tomatoes, diced
3	green onions, chopped
1/4 cup	cilantro, chopped
1 clove	garlic, minced
1/2	yellow bell pepper, diced
1	ripe avocado, diced
1/4 tsp	sea salt
1 tsp	toasted sesame oil (optional)
2-3 tbsp	Herbed Hemp Seed Dressing (recipe on page 96)

DIRECTIONS

1. Soak rice overnight or 8 hours with enough water to cover rice and leave an inch of water. The rice will expand. Start with very warm water.
2. Drain and rinse the rice. Cut collards down the center & cut in half again.
3. Add rice and all other ingredients (except sprouts, collards and dressing) to a bowl and gently stir until all ingredients are well incorporated.
4. Spoon rice mixture onto collard leaf and top with sprouts and dressing and serve. Can be served cold or slightly warmed.

SERVINGS	TIME	LEVEL	KCAL	FIBER	CARB	FAT	PROTEIN
4	25 mins	easy	324	6g	32g	20g	9g

Creamy Raw Collard Greens

This is one of my favorite and relatively, simple recipes. A big bowl of these greens can be a great dinner or lunch!

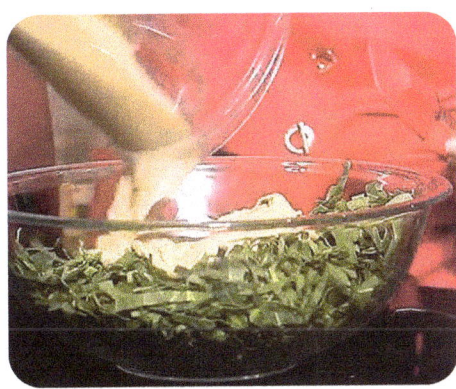

Collard greens are rich in vitamins A, C, K and calcium, supporting immunity and bone health.

INGREDIENTS

2 small	bunches organic collard greens, thinly chopped, stems removed
1 large	avocado, diced
1 large	tomato, diced

Dressing Ingredients

1 cup	raw almonds, soaked for 2-24 hours, drained
1	yellow or red bell pepper
3 cloves	garlic
1	lime, peeled
1 tsp	cayenne pepper (add ½ to 1 tsp more for spicy greens)
1/2 tbsp	chili powder
2 tbsp	tamari
1/4 cup	water (as needed)

DIRECTIONS

1. Gently massage greens in a bowl for 1 minute to tenderize. Blend all dressing ingredients in blender until smooth.
2. Pour dressing over sliced collard greens and mix until greens are fully coated.
3. Add diced tomato and avocado and gently mix until tomatoes and avocado are well distributed.
4. Serve immediately or refrigerate. This recipes works best with a high powered blender such as a Vitamix or Ninja.

SERVINGS	TIME	LEVEL	KCAL	FIBER	CARB	FAT	PROTEIN
3	25 mins	easy	475	16g	32g	36g	18g

Quick Smoky Collards

Yes, collard greens can taste delicious without meat! This is a quick version of collards that retain some of the green's crispness.

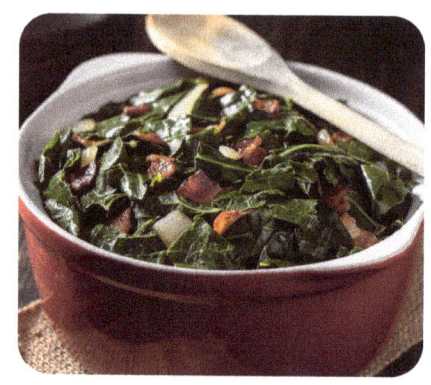

Tomatoes, including sun-dried tomatoes, reduce the risk of certain cancers, like prostate, breast, and lung cancer.

INGREDIENTS

1 pound	collard greens, washed and de-stemmed, cut into 1/2 inch ribbons
½ cup	organic vegetable broth
1	yellow or white onion, diced small
7 cloves	garlic, minced
1 tbsp	smoked paprika
1 tbsp	tamari
1 tsp	liquid smoke
1 tsp	apple cider vinegar
1/2 tsp	Sriracha
1/2 tsp	sea salt
1/4 tsp	cayenne pepper
1/2 cup	sundried tomatoes, chopped

DIRECTIONS

1. Add 2 -3 tablespoons of vegetable broth, onions and garlic to a large sauce pan and saute over medium heat for 4-5 minutes.
2. Add remaining vegetable stock, collard greens and all other ingredients. Cook for 12-15 minutes until greens are softened but bright green. Add water as needed to keep a small amount of liquid in sauce pan.
3. Add sundried tomatoes and stir.
4. Remove from heat and serve.

SERVINGS	TIME	LEVEL	KCAL	FIBER	CARB	FAT	PROTEIN
3	20 mins	easy	44	2g	8g	1g	3g

Cashew Cream Sauce and Zucchini Pasta

Raw zucchini is the best way to eat zucchini! You never have to worry about "over cooked" pasta with this dish.

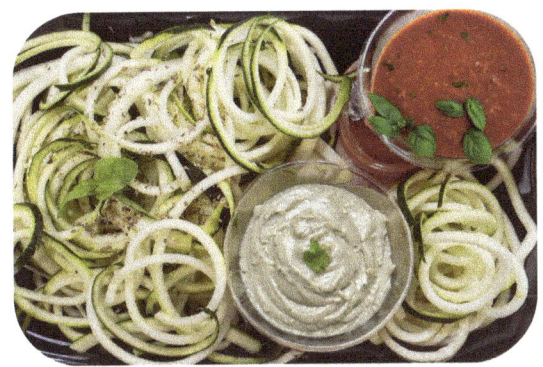

Cashews are rich in zinc & antioxidants, which help strengthen the immune system and support wound healing.

INGREDIENTS

2 large	zucchinis, washed
1/2 cup	raw cashews
1/2 cup	nutritional yeast
1	lemon, juiced
1/2 tsp	sea salt
1/4 cup	fresh basil
2-3	sundried tomatoes
3 cloves	garlic
1 tbsp	tamari
1/2 cup	water, adjust to desired thickness

DIRECTIONS

1. Spiralize 2 zucchinis (skin on) with a spiralizer or mandolin.
2. Optional: soak cashews in water for 2 to 24 hours. Drain right before use. This makes blending easier and the nuts easier to digest.
3. Blend all ingredients together (except zucchinis) in a high-speed blender until smooth.
4. Add enough water to mixture to keep blender moving.
5. Mixture should be thick, but slightly pourable.
6. Pour sauce over the zucchini and serve.
7. Warm gently, but avoid boiling.

SERVINGS	TIME	LEVEL	KCAL	FIBER	CARB	FAT	PROTEIN
2-3	30 mins	Medium	409	7g	33g	26g	20g

Pistachio Pesto with Zucchini Pasta

Zucchini noodles work raw or lightly sautéed, perfect for salads, stir-fries, or cold pasta dishes.

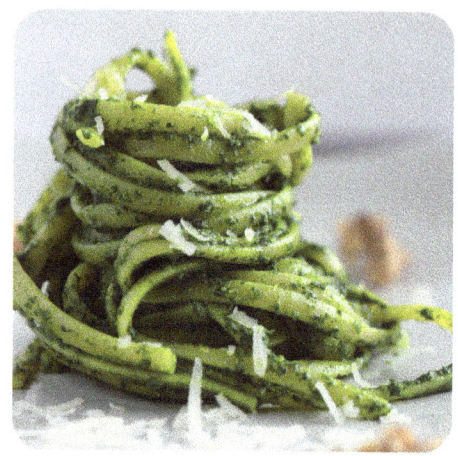

Pistachios are full of antioxidants, healthy fats, and vitamin B6, boosting immunity and reducing inflammation.

INGREDIENTS

2 cups	fresh basil, lightly packed
1.5 cup	pistachios
1/2 cup	nutritional yeast
2 tbsp	lemon juice
1/2 tsp	sea salt
5 cloves	garlic
1/4 tbsp	cracked pepper
3 tbsp	tamari
¼ cup	water to loosen mixture if needed

Pasta: 2 large zucchinis, organic

DIRECTIONS

1. Wash and spiralize raw zucchinis (skin on) with a spiralizer or mandolin.
2. Pulse all ingredients together (except zucchinis) in a food processor until well chopped and mixed.
3. Add a little water to the mix if needed. Add a tablespoon at a time.
4. Spoon the pesto over the zucchini and serve!

SERVINGS	TIME	LEVEL	KCAL	FIBER	CARB	FAT	PROTEIN
3	25 mins	Medium	487	13g	34g	29g	28g

Almond Garlic Pesto

This was a go-to dish during my cancer recovery. I added lots more garlic though!
Serve on toast, with pita bread, with veggies or tossed over pasta.

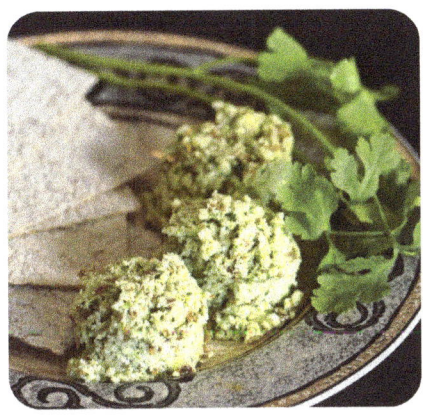

INGREDIENTS

1/2 cup	raw almonds
1 cup	fresh cilantro (parsley also works)
2 tbsp	lemon juice, fresh squeezed
1-2 tbsp	virgin olive oil (optional)
4 cloves	raw garlic (or more to taste)

Cilantro is packed with antioxidants that help detoxify the body. Garlic's sulfur compounds (like allicin) may help protect against certain cancers by blocking cell damage and slowing tumor growth—studies show it's especially promising for stomach and colon cancers.

DIRECTIONS

1. Add all ingredients to a food processor except the olive oil.
2. Pulse the food processor until all ingredients are combined.
3. While the processor is running add the olive oil a tablespoon at a time until the desired consistency is reached.
4. Serve immediately or store in the refrigerator up to 5 days.

SERVINGS	TIME	LEVEL	KCAL	FIBER	CARB	FAT	PROTEIN
2	15 mins	Easy	488	9g	19g	43g	16g

No-Mayo Zesty Dill Coleslaw

A crisp, no-mayo slaw. Yes, it has raisins (but trust me)! The combo of sweet raisins (takes the place of traditionally used sugar), tangy mustard, fresh dill, and crunchy veggies just works.

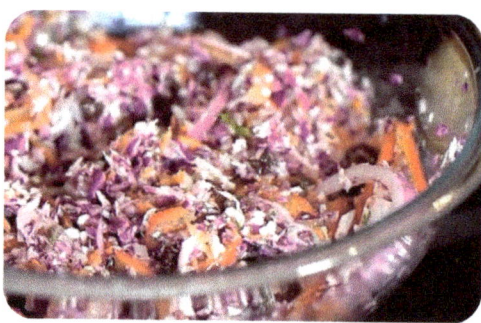

Green cabbage is rich in vitamin K and sulforaphane, a compound studied for its potential to protect cells from damage.

INGREDIENTS

Dressing

1/3 cup	extra virgin cold pressed olive oil
1/4 cup	apple cider vinegar
2/3 cup	raisins
1.5 tsp	sea salt
3 tbsp	prepared mustard
1/3 cup	fresh dill weed, chopped

Slaw

1/2 head	green cabbage, shredded
1/2 head	purple cabbage
1 large	carrot grated
1	red onion, thinly sliced
1	red or yellow bell peppers, thinly sliced

DIRECTIONS

1. Mix dressing ingredients together with a whisk.
2. Pour dressing over salad and mix thoroughly.
3. Serve immediately or chill in refrigerator for a few hours – its best chilled for at least 1 hour.

SERVINGS	TIME	LEVEL	KCAL	FIBER	CARB	FAT	PROTEIN
6-10	25 mins	easy	303	9g	34g	19g	5g

Easy Creamy Coleslaw

In this coleslaw recipe, the apple brings the sweetness and the radish adds a little kick.

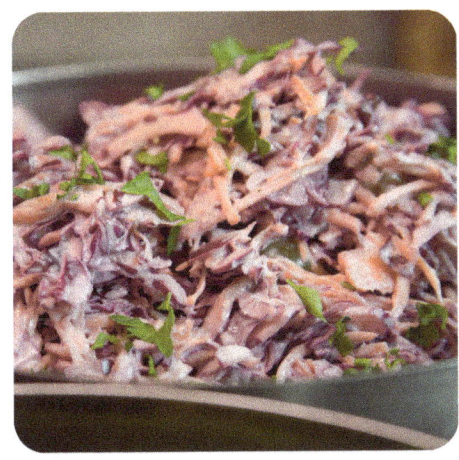

Purple cabbage's deep color comes from anthocyanins, antioxidants linked to heart health and sharper memory. Bonus: It has twice the vitamin C of green cabbage.

INGREDIENTS

1 cup	Creamy Poppy Seed Dressing (recipe on page 95)
½ head	green cabbage, shredded
½ head	purple cabbage, shredded
1 large	carrot, grated
4	radishes, grated
1	zucchini, grated
1	organic red apple, grated

DIRECTIONS

1. Grate all vegetables with a food processor or hand grater.
2. Pour dressing over veggies and mix well. Serve immediately or let chill for 30 minutes.

SERVINGS	TIME	LEVEL	KCAL	FIBER	CARB	FAT	PROTEIN
8-10	25 mins	easy	171	8g	28g	6g	5g

Lemon Asparagus with Cotija "Cheese"

This simple recipe sings with flavor and brings together several foods that boost the immune system, help reduce inflammation and are high in anti-oxidants, eat up!

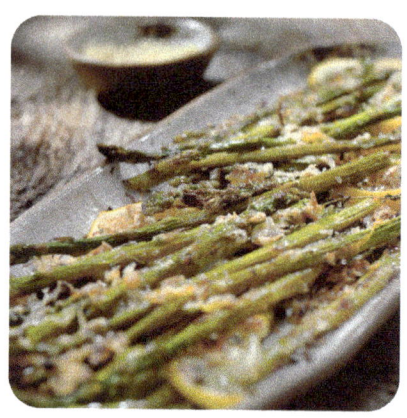

INGREDIENTS

20	stalks of asparagus (1.5 pounds)
1 cup	cremini or shitake mushrooms, chopped
1/4 cup	Vegan Cotija Cheese (recipe on the page 106)
2 tbsp	lemon juice, fresh squeezed
1 tbsp	lemon zest (use organic lemons)
1/2 tsp	sea salt

Asparagus is packed with antioxidants like vitamin C and glutathione, which help strengthen the immune system and fight off harmful free radicals!

DIRECTIONS

1. Cut off the bottom inch off the asparagus stalk. Chop asparagus into 2-inch pieces. Cut the asparagus on the bias (at an angle).
2. Sauté chopped asparagus and mushrooms over medium heat with a 2-4 tablespoons of water for 5-6 minutes.
3. Add lemon juice and zest of 1 organic lemon and sprinkle with sea salt and saute for another 2-3 minutes. Asparagus should be bright green with a little firmness.
4. Remove from heat and sprinkle with cojita. Mix well and top with additional tablespoon of cojita. Serve immediately.

SERVINGS	TIME	LEVEL	KCAL	FIBER	CARB	FAT	PROTEIN
3	20 mins	easy	159	5g	10g	12g	7g

Maple Mustard Brussels Sprouts

This recipe turns cruciferous veggies (the ones filled with sulforaphane) into the best bite on the plate.

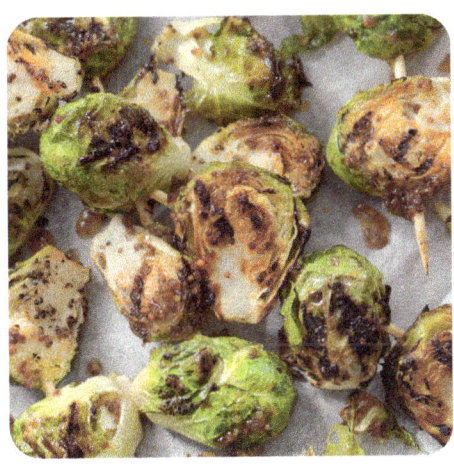

INGREDIENTS

1 pound	Brussels sprouts
2 tbsp	pure maple syrup
1 tbsp	coconut oil (optional)
1 tbsp	brown mustard
1/4 tsp	sea salt and cracked pepper
dash	cayenne pepper
2	garlic cloves

Brussels sprouts are rich in vitamin C and sulforaphane, powerful compounds that help fight inflammation and boost immune function.

DIRECTIONS

1. Preheat oven to 400°F.
2. Wash and cut brussels in half and remove any brown outer leaves.
3. Mix mustard, maple syrup, salt/pepper and cayenne together, in a small bowl with a whisk.
4. Coat the Brussels with the marinade.
5. Place the Brussels on an oiled cookie sheet or a cookie sheet lined with parchment.
6. Roast in oven for about 30 minute. Stir half way through and add crushed garlic.

SERVINGS	TIME	LEVEL	KCAL	FIBER	CARB	FAT	PROTEIN
2	40 mins	easy	176	3g	20g	11g	2g

Roasted Brussels Sprouts with Cherry Tomatoes

The tomatoes in this dish add a delicious sweet burst of flavor!

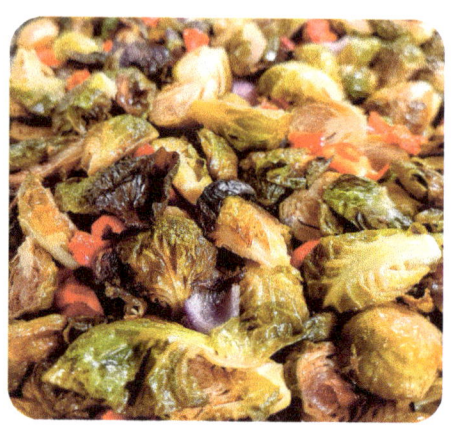

INGREDIENTS

1.5 pounds	Brussels sprouts
1 tbsp	extra virgin olive oil
3 tbsp	balsamic vinegar
3/4 tsp	sea salt
1/2 tsp	freshly ground black pepper
1 pint	cherry tomatoes

Cooked tomatoes have increased levels of lycopene which have the protective effect of neutralizing free radicals that contribute to cancer development.

DIRECTIONS

1. Preheat the oven to 350°F.
2. Cut off the ends of the Brussels and pull off any yellow outer leaves.
3. Mix them in a bowl with the olive oil, balsamic vinegar, salt, and pepper.
4. Turn them out on an oiled baking sheet and roast for 30 minutes. Reserve remaining olive oil and balsamic vinegar mixture.
5. Cut cherry tomatoes in half and mix with remaining mixture.
6. Remove pan from oven and place tomatoes on the pan with the sprouts.
7. Bake for another 15-20 minutes, until sprouts are crisp outside and tender inside.
8. Shake the pan from time to time, to brown the Brussels sprouts evenly. Sprinkle with more sea salt and serve.

SERVINGS	TIME	LEVEL	KCAL	FIBER	CARB	FAT	PROTEIN
3	20 mins	easy	73	3g	10g	3g	3g

Rosemary and Garlic Roasted Cauliflower

More cruciferous veggies! This serves an easy side dish or even as an afternoon snack.

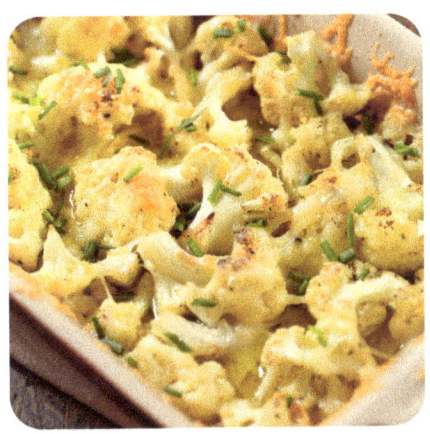

Cauliflower is loaded with vitamin C and sulforaphane, powerful compounds that enhance immunity and fight disease.

INGREDIENTS

1 head	cauliflower, washed, cut into florets
10 cloves	garlic, minced
1/4 cup	coconut or olive oil
1.5 tbsp	dried rosemary
1 tsp	sea salt
Dash	cracked pepper, to taste

DIRECTIONS

1. Preheat oven to 400°F.
2. Mix oil, rosemary, salt, pepper and garlic together in a large bowl.
3. Toss cauliflower into bowl and mix until cauliflower is coated.
4. Place flat into large baking dish or pan.
5. Bake for 35-40 minutes until lightly browned; stir occasionally.
6. Serve immediately.

SERVINGS	TIME	LEVEL	KCAL	FIBER	CARB	FAT	PROTEIN
3	45 mins	easy	115	2g	7g	9g	2g

Savory Sweet Potato & Roasted Mushrooms

Sweet potatoes, but savory: roasted mushrooms turn this into a hearty, unexpected win.

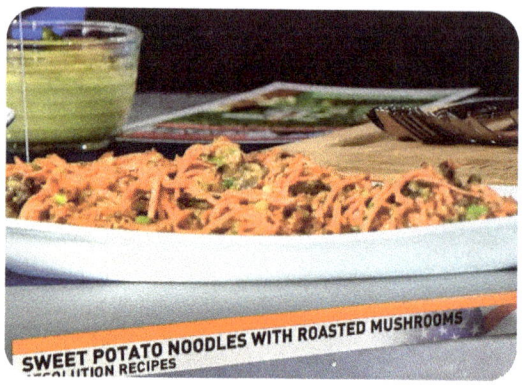

SWEET POTATO NOODLES WITH ROASTED MUSHROOMS
REVOLUTION RECIPES

Sweet potatoes are rich in beta-carotene, which supports eye health and boosts immunity.

INGREDIENTS

2 med	sweet potatoes
2 cups	cremini mushrooms
3/4 cup	tahini
1/4 cup	white miso paste
1/2 cup	tamari, plus 2 tbsp
3 tbsp	lemon juice
4 tbsp	stone ground brown mustard
2 tbsp	maple syrup
1 bunch	green onions, chopped
1/2 cup	hemp seeds

DIRECTIONS

1. Preheat oven to 450°F.
2. Slice mushrooms and marinate with 2 tablespoons tamari. Place on baking sheet and let bake for 15-20 minutes.
3. Wash, peel & shred raw sweet potatoes with a food processor or manual shredder. Alternatively you could use a tabletop spiralizer and spiralize the sweet potatoes.
4. Place tahini, tamari, lemon juice, mustard and maple syrup in a bowl and whisk until well incorporated.
5. Pour sauce over sweet potatoes and mix. Sauté in a pan on medium heat for 5-7 minutes.
6. Add mushrooms, chopped green onions and hemp seeds and mix well. Enjoy!

SERVINGS	TIME	LEVEL	KCAL	FIBER	CARB	FAT	PROTEIN
3	20 mins	easy	434	5g	29g	31g	16g

Raw Celeriac (Celery Root) Soup

You can find celery root at many health foods stores near root vegetables like turnips and parsnips.

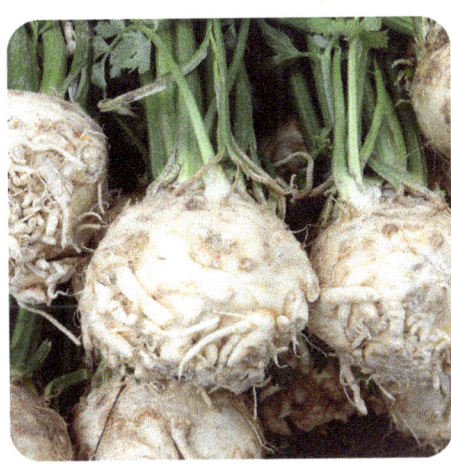

Raw celery root (celeriac) has a crisp texture and a mild, earthy flavor with hints of celery and parsley.

INGREDIENTS

1 med	celery root (5 cups peeled & cubed, 2-3 inches)
2 tbsp	coconut oil
2 tbsp	olive oil
1.5 cups	raw cashews, soaked 1 hour or more, drained
2 cups	water
1 cup	almond or coconut milk (unsweetened)
3 tbsp	nutritional yeast
5 cloves	garlic
1 tsp	sea salt
1 tsp	chicken style seasoning (optional)
1/2 tsp	cayenne pepper
1 tsp	Bell's Seasoning (rosemary, oregano, sage, ginger, marjoram, thyme, & pepper
1 large	avocado, diced (garnish)
1/2 cup	leeks, thinly sliced (garnish)

DIRECTIONS

1. Add water and celery root to blender and blend until almost smooth.
2. Add all other ingredients besides avocado and leeks and blend until smooth (if using a VitaMix, blend until slightly warm).
3. Pour soup into bowls, top with diced avocado and leeks, and serve.

SERVINGS	TIME	LEVEL	KCAL	FIBER	CARB	FAT	PROTEIN
4	20 mins	easy	462	9g	36g	33g	14g

Raw Corn Chowder

A no-cook, creamy soup that's surprisingly rich and satisfying.

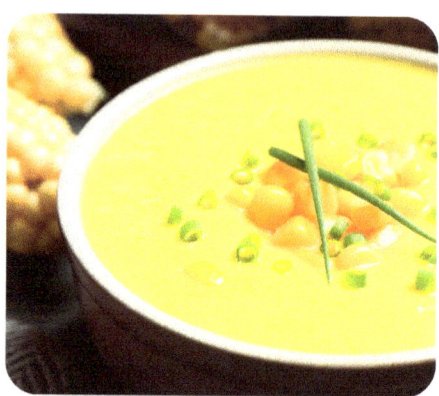

Raw corn retains more vitamin C. It also has a higher water content, making it extra hydrating.

INGREDIENTS

2.5 cup	sweet corn
1/2 cup	organic cashews
1,5 cup	water
1 cup	coconut water
1	lime, juiced
2 cloves	garlic, peeled
1 tsp	paprika
1/2 tsp	sea salt (or to taste)
Pinch of	cayenne

Optional toppings: cilantro or chopped avocado

DIRECTIONS

1. Place all liquids into the blender and ½ of the corn into a blender and blend until smooth.
2. Slowly add the remaining corn and cashews until smooth. Add additional water for a thinner consistency.
3. If using a high speed blender, such as a Vitamix blender, you may blend until it is slightly warm.
   Note: set some corn aside and add it after blending for more texture.

SERVINGS	TIME	LEVEL	KCAL	FIBER	CARB	FAT	PROTEIN
3	20 mins	easy	600	5g	52g	43g	16g

Creamy Asparagus Soup

As a creamy soup fanatic and asparagus lover, this bowl is my happy place.

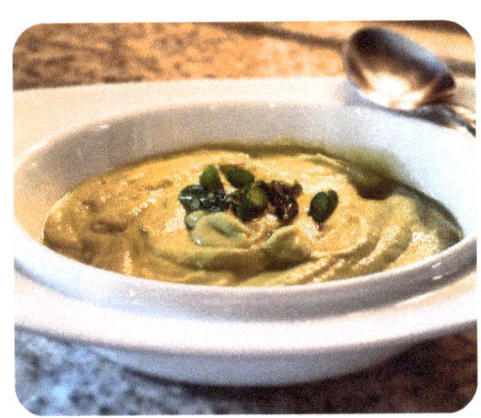

INGREDIENTS

8 stalks	asparagus (about ½ a bunch)
3/4 cup	raw cashews
1 tbsp	lemon juice
1 tbsp	coconut aminos or tamari
2 cloves	garlic
Dash	cracked pepper
½ tsp	sea salt
1.5 cups	water

Asparagus is rich in vitamin C, vitamin E, and glutathione, a powerful antioxidant that helps protect immune cells from damage. It also contains prebiotic fiber, which supports gut health, a key component of a strong immune system. 🌿

DIRECTIONS

1. Preheat oven to 400°F.
2. Cut off the bottom inch off the asparagus and discard.
3. Pace asparagus on a cookie sheet and spray a spritz of olive oil. Roast in over for 10 minutes. Remove from oven.
4. Place all ingredients into a blender and blend until smooth.
5. Slowly add additional water for a thinner consistency, if desired.

SERVINGS	TIME	LEVEL	KCAL	FIBER	CARB	FAT	PROTEIN
2-4	25 mins	easy	284	3g	22g	20g	10g

Fire-Roasted Tomato Basil Soup

Warm, comforting, and seriously good! Serve with crispy roasted chickpeas or croutons to add crunch and take it up a notch.

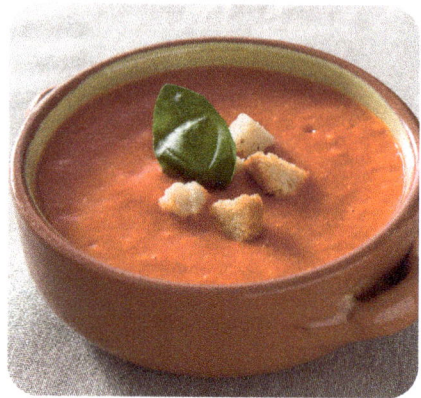

Lycopene, an antioxidant in tomatoes, supports heart health by lowering blood pressure & cholesterol, and protecting cells from oxidative damage.

INGREDIENTS

2	ripe tomatoes, chopped
56 oz	canned fire-roasted tomatoes
2 large	carrots, chopped
1 cup	fresh basil, chiffonade
1 cup	coconut milk
1/2 cup	vegetable broth
1	onion, chopped
3 cloves	garlic, crushed
1 tsp	dried oregano
1/2 tsp	sea salt
¼ tsp	black pepper, or to taste

DIRECTIONS

1. Add 2-3 tablespoons water or vegetable broth, onion and garlic to a pot and sauté until softened. Then add the oregano, dried basil, carrots, fire-roasted tomatoes and fresh tomatoes and mix together.
2. Add in the vegetable stock and bring to the boil. Turn down the heat, cover the pot and leave to simmer until the carrots are softened.
3. Remove from the heat and stir in the fresh basil and coconut milk. Blend with an immersion blender or by transferring to your blender jug in stages and then returning to the pot. Add salt and pepper to taste.

SERVINGS	TIME	LEVEL	KCAL	FIBER	CARB	FAT	PROTEIN
3	25 mins	easy	455	12g	51g	28g	11g

Spring Rolls with Spicy Peanut Dipping Sauce

To make the best spring rolls, use your favorite fresh ingredients! Below are a few of mine.

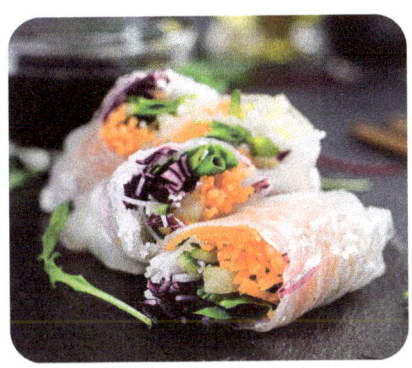

Rice paper wraps keep these spring rolls light, while the peanut sauce delivers protein and a kick of heat.

FILLING INGREDIENTS:

6-8	rice paper sheets
1 cup	baby spinach
2	carrots, spiralized
1	cucumber, sliced into spears
4 large	portobello mushrooms, sliced (marinated in tamari)
1/2	red, yellow or orange bell pepper, thinly sliced
½ cup	basil, (2-3 leaves per roll)
¼ cup	raw cashews (sprinkle a few in each roll)

Peanut Dipping Sauce:

2 tbsp	peanut butter
2-3 tbsp	grated fresh ginger
4 tbsp	brown rice vinegar
1 tbsp	maple syrup or agave nectar
1/2	jalapeno pepper, seeded (use the whole pepper to make it spicier)
¼ - ½ cup	water (more or less to get desired consistency)

DIRECTIONS

Dipping Sauce:

Put all sauce ingredients in a blender and blend until creamy.
Set aside.

Continued on the next page.

SERVINGS	TIME	LEVEL	KCAL	FIBER	CARB	FAT	PROTEIN
3	20 mins	Intermediate	530	6g	47g	16g	13g

Spring Rolls with Spicy Peanut Dipping Sauce

The peanut sauce is really the show stopper, so good!

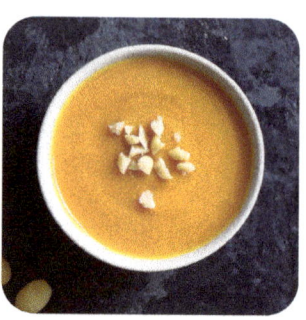

Peanuts are a great source of protein, healthy fats, and antioxidants like resveratrol, which help improve heart health, support muscle growth, and reduce inflammation.

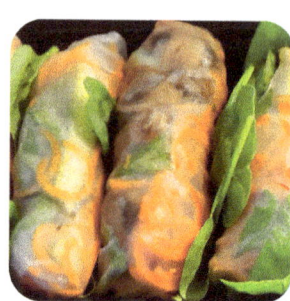

SPRING ROLL DIRECTIONS

1. Fill a pie plate or bowl with hot water. Immerse 1 rice paper in warm water for a 3-5 seconds to soften it up a little (work with one rice paper at a time, being gentle as they break easily). Remove from water and place rice paper on a clean kitchen towel.
2. Arrange a few pieces of spinach on bottom half of rice paper leaving a 1-inch border along edge. Add the rest of the ingredients in any order. Top with some of the mushrooms and basil;(don't overfill). Be sure to evenly distribute the ingredients from one end.
3. Pressing down on the filling with your fingers, fold the bottom end of the sheet (side nearest you) over the top of the fillings and roll into a cylindrical shape halfway.
4. Fold the left and right sides inward and complete rolling the remaining half (If rice paper is too dry to seal, moisten unsealed edges with a little more warm water). Transfer spring roll to a plate, seam-side down, and cover with dampened paper towels. Make additional roll in the same manner.
5. I usually place spinach between the rolls to keep them from sticking together. Serve with dipping sauce.

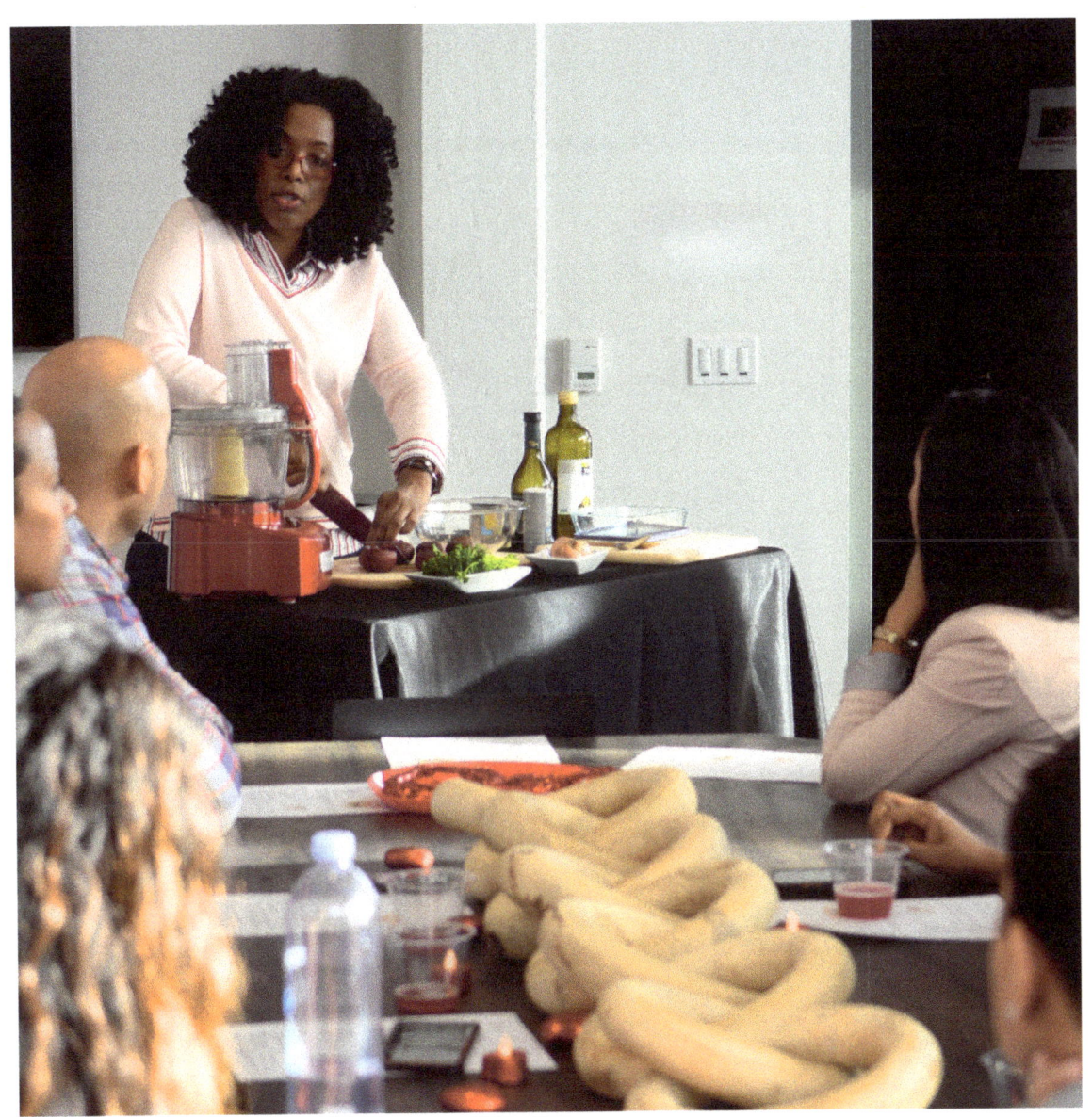

Whipping up some thyroid nourishing goodness!

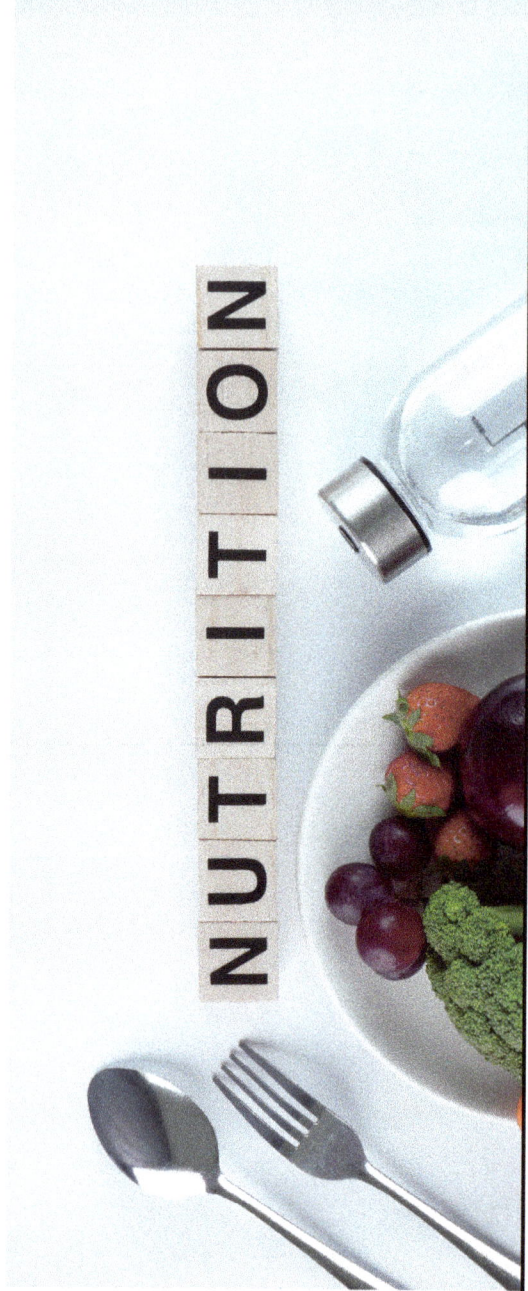

NUTRITION

Eat like your cells are listening. Your thyroid always is.

- 4 -
THYROID NOURISHING

Thyroid Nourishing Recipes

Your thyroid might be small, but it's the quiet conductor of your entire body—energy, metabolism, even mood. And just like any delicate instrument, it thrives on the right fuel. This chapter is about the foods that actually support it: everyday ingredients that shield and strengthen.

I built these recipes to care for your thyroid, Brazil nuts in the hemp milk for selenium, walnuts in the tacos for zinc, and coconut for metabolism-loving fats. My Spiralized Beets & Almond Pesto pulls double duty: basil fights inflammation, beets support detox, and almonds deliver thyroid-critical magnesium and vitamin E. Eating well shouldn't feel like medicine. It should taste so good, you forget it's healing you. These recipes don't force you to choose between flavor and function, they deliver both.

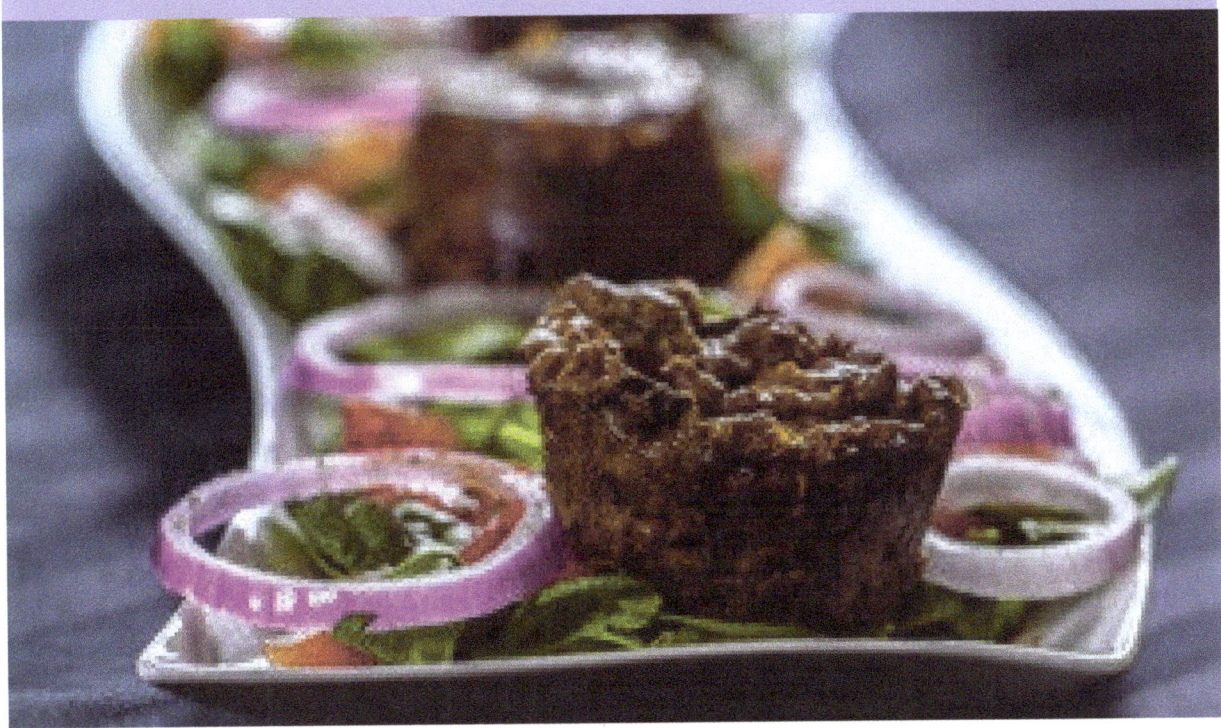

Eggless Quiche

Eggless Coconut 'Egg' Salad

I love to experiment with dishes that are reminiscent of some old favorites. Black salt has sulfur compounds that create an eggy umami effect without the eggs.

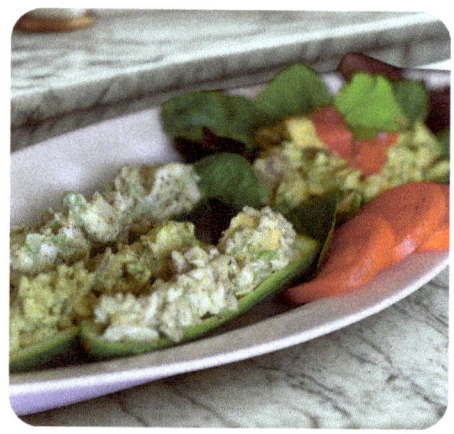

Coconuts contain medium-chain triglycerides (MCTs), a type of fat that is quickly converted into energy, boosting metabolism and supports brain health.

INGREDIENTS

1.5 cup	coconut meat, diced small
1	avocado, peeled, diced large
1	celery stalks, coarsely chopped
1	lemon, juiced
1/2 cup	vegan mayonnaise
1 tbsp	prepared mustard (made w/apple cider vinegar)
1 tbsp	powdered mustard
1.5 tbsp	fresh dill (preferred) or 1 tsp dried dill
1 tsp	celery seed
1/2 tsp	sea salt
1/2 tsp	black salt (highly recommended)
1/4 tsp	turmeric

DIRECTIONS

1. Roughly chop coconut meet into approximately ½ inch pieces.
2. Mix in all ingredients except the avocado until well blended.
3. Taste and adjust seasonings as desired.
4. Gently mix in avocado until well coated. Serve immediately. Keeps up to 3 days, refrigerated.

Serving suggestions: on bed mixed greens, on a gluten-free roll/bun, with sliced red/yellow bell pepper, with raw or gluten-free crackers.

SERVINGS	TIME	LEVEL	KCAL	FIBER	CARB	FAT	PROTEIN
3	20 mins	easy	740	13g	23g	73g	6g

Coconut Avocado Wraps

If you're looking to spend minimal time in the kitchen, this recipe has you covered!

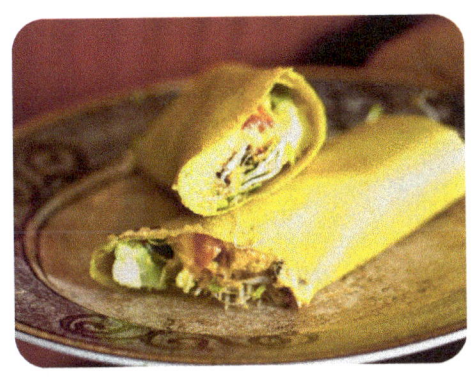

Avocados are one of the few fruits high in monounsaturated fats, which help reduce inflammation and support brain function.

INGREDIENTS

4 raw	coconut wraps (aka as paleo wraps), or whole wheat or gluten free wrap
6 tbsp	hummus
1 cup	alfalfa or broccoli sprouts
1	Roma tomato, sliced
1	avocado, sliced
1/2	red or yellow bell pepper (optional)
1 dash	sea salt
1 tsp	balsamic vinegar

DIRECTIONS

1. Add ¼ of ingredients to each wrap. Drizzle balsamic vinegar over sprouts.
2. Roll the wrap securely and slice.
3. Serve immediately or store in the refrigerator.

SERVINGS	TIME	LEVEL	KCAL	FIBER	CARB	FAT	PROTEIN
3-4	15 mins	easy	279	8g	14g	25g	5g

Goji Almond Hemp Milk

This deliciously healthy treat is packed with thyroid-nourishing ingredients.
Almonds (zinc) + hemp seeds (omega-3s + magnesium).

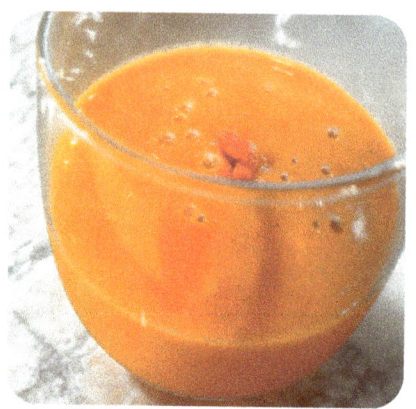

Goji berries are rich in zeaxanthin, an antioxidant that supports eye health.

INGREDIENTS

5 cups	purified water
1 cup	almonds
1/2 cup	goji berries
1/4 cup	hempseeds (optional)
7	pitted Medjool dates (about ¼ cup), omit for an unsweetened version
1/2 tsp	cinnamon
1/4 tsp	sea salt

DIRECTIONS

1. Add all ingredients to a highspeed blender and blend until smooth.
2. Refrigerate for 2 or more hours and serve. Milk will last 5-7 days refrigerated in a glass container, tightly sealed.
3. Shake or stir well before serving, as some settling will occur.

SERVINGS	TIME	LEVEL	KCAL	FIBER	CARB	FAT	PROTEIN
6	15 mins	easy	360	7g	35g	23g	10g

Goji Brazil Hemp Milk

This refreshing drink is delicious on its own or as a base for a smoothie.

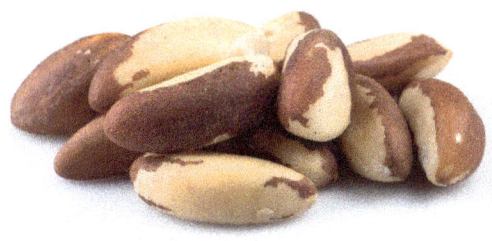

INGREDIENTS

4 cups	purified water
1/4 cup	Brazil nuts
1/2 cup	hempseeds, shelled
1/2 cup	goji berries
7	pitted Medjool dates (¼ cup), omit for an unsweetened version
1/2 tsp	cinnamon (or to taste)
1/4 tsp	sea salt

Brazil nuts are the best source of selenium, which supports thyroid function.

DIRECTIONS

1. Add all ingredients to a highspeed blender and blend until smooth.
2. Refrigerate for 2 or more hours and serve. Milk will last 5-7 days refrigerated in a glass container, tightly sealed.
3. Shake or stir well before serving as some settling will occur.

SERVINGS	TIME	LEVEL	KCAL	FIBER	CARB	FAT	PROTEIN
4-8	15 mins	easy	251	4g	29g	14g	7g

'Must-Try' Mango Chia Seed Pudding

This pudding supports thyroid health with healthy fats, antioxidants, and vitamins and minerals like B6, A, C, and zinc, helping reduce inflammation and balance hormones.

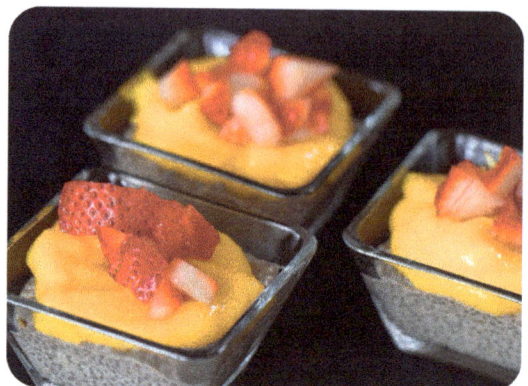

Chia seeds are rich in omega-3s, fiber, and antioxidants, supporting heart health and reducing inflammation

INGREDIENTS

4-5 tbsp	chia seeds
2	bananas
3/4 cup	unsweetened coconut milk
1 tbsp	coconut nectar
1 tsp	vanilla extract
1 tsp	cinnamon
1 tbsp	cardamom
3/4 cup	strawberries, diced
1.5 cups	mango (fresh or frozen), chopped

DIRECTIONS

1. Peel and mash bananas well with a fork in a bowl.
2. Add chia seeds to the banana mash and mix well.
3. Add in coconut milk, vanilla, cinnamon, and cardamom to chia seed mash. Whisk until well mixed and mixture becomes thick (about 1 minute). Set aside in refrigerator to set for at least 1 hour to overnight. Alternative: for a creamier pudding, add chia mix to a blender and blend until smooth. Let set.
4. Add mango to blender and puree. Add 1 or 2 tablespoons of water if needed to get blender moving. Puree should be thick
5. Top chia pudding evenly with mango puree, Top with diced kiwi. Alternatively, separate chia pudding into 4-6 even portions. Top with mango puree and kiwi.
6. Serve for refrigerate pudding, tightly covered, up to 4 days.

SERVINGS	TIME	LEVEL	KCAL	FIBER	CARB	FAT	PROTEIN
4-6	20-60 mins	easy	267	9g	34g	15g	5g

10-Minute Raw Tacos

This dish gets requested, a lot! I love easy raw recipes; they're forgiving, quick to prepare (soaking aside), and nearly impossible to ruin.

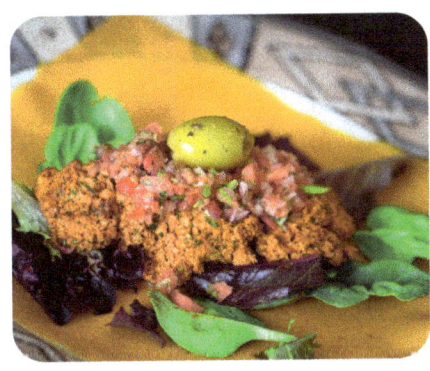

Walnuts are the only nuts rich in plant-based omega-3s, supporting brain and heart health.

INGREDIENTS

1 cup	raw walnuts (soaked for 2 hours, drained
1 small	shallot or 1/2 medium red onion
3/4 cup	sundried tomatoes (oil packed or dehydrated)
1/2	cucumber
1	lime, juiced
3/4 cup	fresh cilantro
2 tsp	chili powder
1.5 tsp	cumin
1 ½ tsp	Spanish or smoked paprika
1/2 tsp	cayenne pepper
1/2 tsp	sea salt or to taste
1 cup	mixed greens
3-4 tbsp	water to get mixture moving
6	Spanish olives
4	coconut wraps (AKA: paleo wraps), cut in half or 4-5 Blue Corn Taco Shells

DIRECTIONS

1. Put walnuts, cucumber, sundried tomatoes (*do not substitute this*), lime, cilantro, and seasonings, into a food processor and pulse until ingredients are incorporated.
2. Stop in between to scrape down sides. Add a tablespoon of water as needed. Mixture should be thick and have the consistency of ground beef.
3. Place coconut wrap (pressed coconut fleshed) or taco shell on plate top with lettuce, add 2-3 tablespoons walnut taco mix; top with salsa (see *Quick & Easy Salsa on the next page*) and a green olive. Alternatives: Serve in an organic taco shell, with vegan sour cream (on page 104).

SERVINGS	TIME	LEVEL	KCAL	FIBER	CARB	FAT	PROTEIN
4-5	10 mins	easy	412	7g	21g	36g	10g

Quick & Easy Salsa

This salsa isn't just perfect for the 10-Minute Raw Tacos—it also adds amazing flavor to avocado toast, baked potatoes, and scrambled tofu.

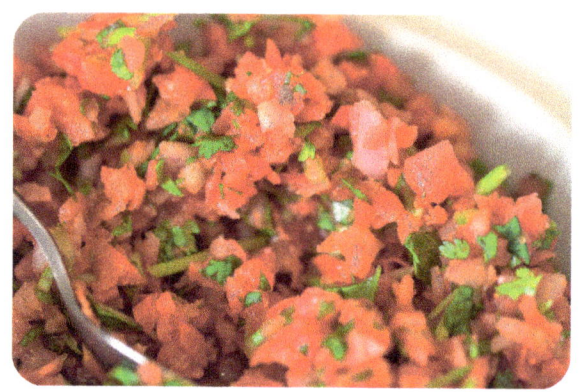

A natural detoxifier, cilantro helps remove heavy metals from the body while adding a fresh, zesty flavor.

INGREDIENTS

2 med	tomatoes
3/4 cup	fresh cilantro
1/2 med	onion
1	lime, juiced
1.5 tsp	cumin
1/2 tsp	cayenne pepper
1/2 tsp	sea salt or to taste

DIRECTIONS

1. Put all ingredients into a food processor and pulse until ingredients are incorporated but chunky.
2. For extra spicy salsa add ½ or whole jalapeño pepper with seeds.
3. Serve with *10-Minute Raw Tacos*.

SERVINGS	TIME	LEVEL	KCAL	FIBER	CARB	FAT	PROTEIN
4-5	10 mins	easy	16	1g	3g	0	1g

Spaghetti Squash 'Pasta' with Marinara

A raw, no-cook wonder: spaghetti squash 'pasta' meets zesty marinara, light, fresh, and effortlessly delicious!

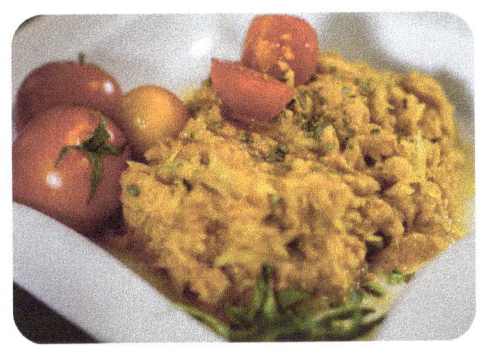

Spaghetti squash is rich in fiber and vitamin C, yet has just a fraction of the carbs of traditional pasta!

SQUASH INGREDIENTS:

1	medium/large spaghetti squash
2 cloves	garlic, crushed
1/2 tsp	sea salt

MARINARA SAUCE INGREDIENTS:

1 cup	sundried tomatoes (in olive oil – include 3 tbsp of the olive oil)
3	medium-large Roma tomatoes
1 ½ tsp	oregano (or 1/8 cup fresh oregano)
1 ½ tsp	basil (or 1/4 cup fresh basil)
3 tbsp	nutritional yeast
1/2 tsp	sea salt
4 cloves	garlic
1	small shallot
1 ½	Medjool dates
3 tbsp	water

Continued on the next page.

SERVINGS	TIME	LEVEL	KCAL	FIBER	CARB	FAT	PROTEIN
2-4	20 mins	easy	214	9g	40g	6g	7g

SQUASH PREPARATION:

1. Cut squash in half and remove seeds. Cut squash into 4-8 pieces. Use a knife or vegetable peeler to remove rind.
2. Julianne squash with a mandolin to shred it using 1/8 inch thickness. Alternatively use a shredding blade in a food processor to shred.
3. Drain squash if needed. Add squash seasonings to squash and mix; set aside.

SAUCE PREPARATION:

1. Add all sauce ingredients to blender except water, and blend until somewhat smooth.
2. Add water as needed.

PUTTING IT TOGETHER:

Pour sauce mixture over spaghetti squash and mix well. Serve & Enjoy!

COOKED SQUASH VERSION:

1. Cut spaghetti squash in half and remove seeds. Bake cut side down for 30-40 minutes at 375°F.
2. Let cool and use fork to scrape out squash.
3. prepare sauce as described above.
4. Gently heat sauce, do not bring to boil. Spoon sauce over squash and serve.

Spiralized Beets with Basil Pesto

This thyroid-nourishing raw recipe features enzyme-rich beets—aiding liver detox, hormone balance, and inflammation—paired with DNA-protecting basil.

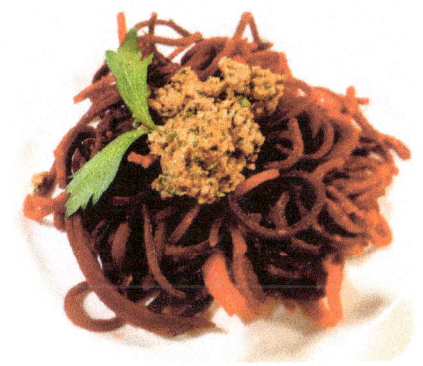

Beets contain betalains, unique antioxidants that fight inflammation and give beets their rich color.

INGREDIENTS

3 med	beets, peeled and spiralized
1 cup	raw almonds
1 cup	fresh basil, packed
1/2	orange bell pepper, seeded
3 tbsp	nutritional yeast
2 tbsp	fresh squeezed lemon juice
4 cloves	garlic (or more to taste)
1/2 tsp	sea salt (to taste)
2-4 tbsp	of water to loosen mixture, if needed

DIRECTIONS

1. Wash and peel beets with a vegetable peeler; spiralize beets with a spiralizer. Best to use a countertop spiralizer for beets. A handheld spiralizer works best for slim, oblong items like zucchini. Set spiralized beets aside.
2. Add all other ingredients to a food processor, except the water.
3. Pulse the food processor until all ingredients are combined.
4. Add a few tablespoons of water if needed and pulse food processor.
5. Place 1/3 of beets on a serving dish and top with 2 scoops of basil pesto.
6. Serve immediately or store in the refrigerator for up to 7 days.

SERVINGS	TIME	LEVEL	KCAL	FIBER	CARB	FAT	PROTEIN
3	20 mins	easy	368	11g	25g	24g	17g

Sunflower Tuna Salad

A fish-free twist! Raw sunflower seeds mimic tuna's texture, loaded with protein, crunch, and zingy flavor. The seaweed adds a mild ocean flavor.

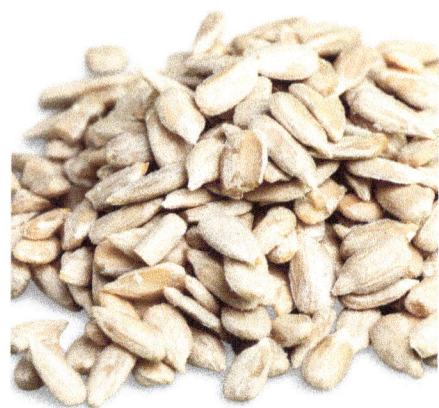

Packed with immune-boosting vitamin E, zinc and selenium.

INGREDIENTS

2 cups	sunflower seeds, soaked 2 hours to overnight
3 tbsp	parsley, chopped
2	cloves garlic
1/2	medium red onion
2	stalks celery
3 tbsp	dulse (seaweed)
2 tbsp	apple cider vinegar
2 tbsp	fresh lemon juice
¾ tsp	sea salt
1 ½ tbsp	brown or Dijon mustard
3 tbsp	vegan mayo
1	diced tomato, finely chopped
2	medium kosher dill pickles

DIRECTIONS

1. Drain and rinse sunflower seeds.
2. Finely chop parsley, onion, and celery or pulse in a food processor; set aside.
3. Mix dulse with apple cider vinegar and lemon juice in a small bowl.
4. Add sunflower seeds, garlic, dulse mixture, mustard, sea salt to food processor. Pulse until seeds are grounded and ingredients are well incorporated.
5. Combine sunflower seed mixture with parsley, onions, celery & vegan mayo in a bowl. Gently mix in diced tomatoes. Serve.

Serving Suggestions: Wrap in romaine lettuce leaves or use as a dip for veggies such as red pepper slices or celery. Serve on a bed of mixed greens or with a side of raw crackers. Serve on toasted whole grain bread with lettuce and tomatoes.

SERVINGS	TIME	LEVEL	KCAL	FIBER	CARB	FAT	PROTEIN
4	25 mins	easy	469	8g	20g	40g	16g

Baked Broccoli Tree Dippers & Cashew Dip

This is a great snack for kids and adults. It can also be served as a side dish. The cashew dip is very versatile and can do double duty as a salad dressing.

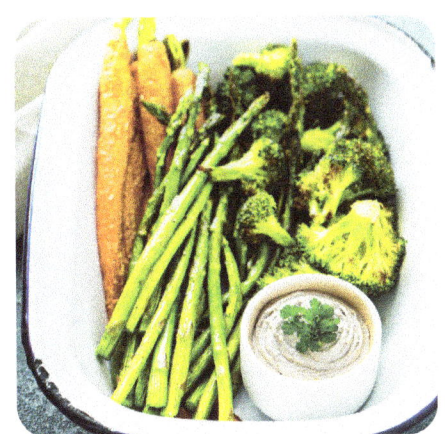

Broccoli's sulforaphane—a potent cancer-fighting compound—also supercharges immunity and cellular defense.

INGREDIENTS

1 bunch	broccoli crowns, sliced/broken into bite size pieces
1/2 tsp	olive oil spray
1 tsp	smoked paprika
1 tsp	garlic powder
1/4 tsp	sea salt

Dip Ingredients

3/4 cup	raw cashews, soaked 2 hours or more, drained
1/2	yellow bell pepper, seeded
1	lemon, juiced (about 2 tbsp)
2 cloves	garlic
1 tbsp	tamari
1 tsp	sea salt, smoked paprika
3/4 cup	water

DIRECTIONS

1. Preheat oven to 375°F.
2. Toss broccoli with olive oil spray, paprika, garlic powder and sea salt until coated.
3. Place on cookie sheet and bake for 30 minutes.
4. While broccoli is baking, add all dip ingredients to a blender. Blend until smooth. Add more water for a thinner consistency.
5. Remove broccoli from oven and let cool for 5 min. Serve broccoli with dip.

SERVINGS	TIME	LEVEL	KCAL	FIBER	CARB	FAT	PROTEIN
3	40 mins	easy	358	8g	33g	22g	15g

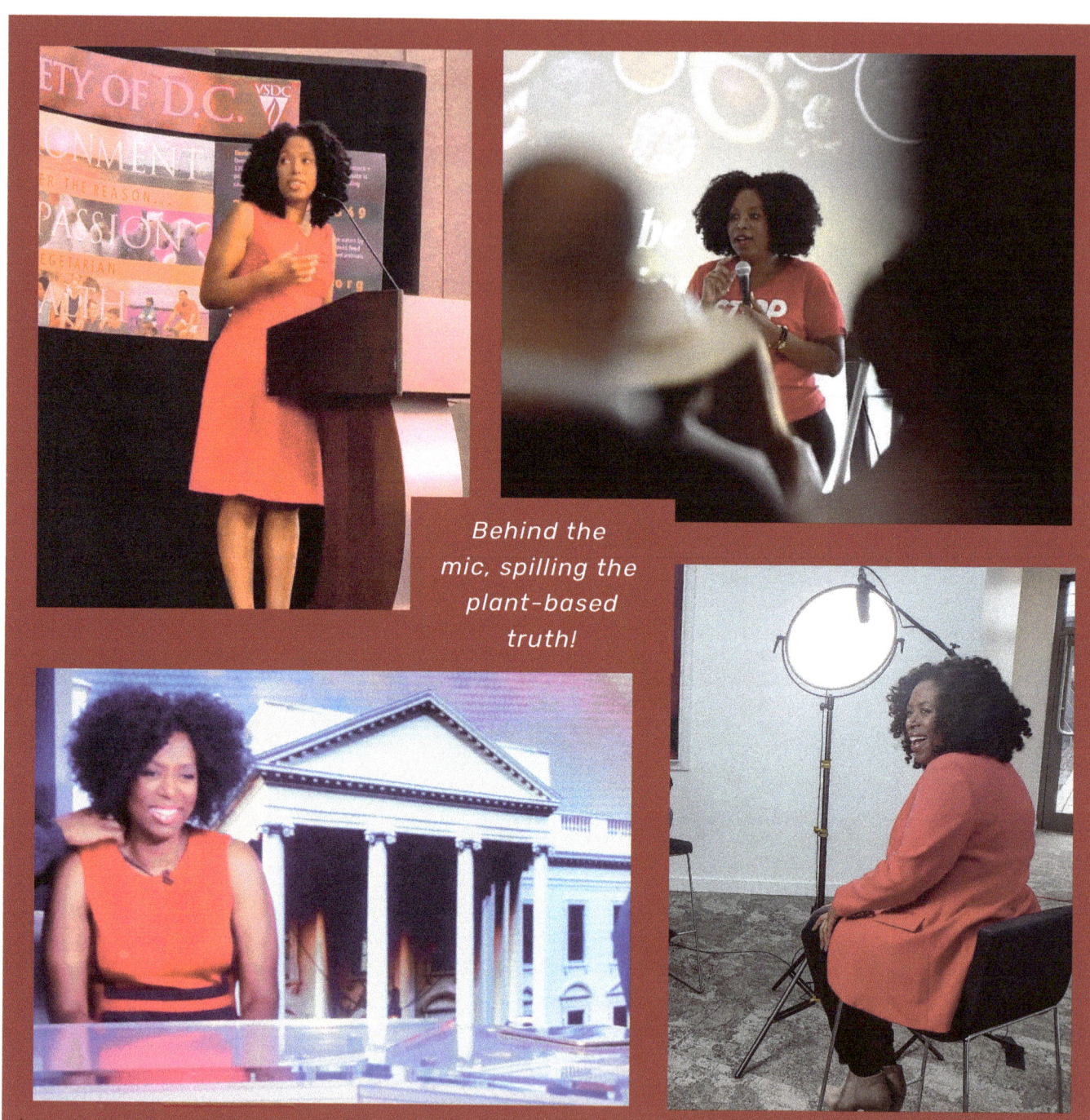

Behind the mic, spilling the plant-based truth!

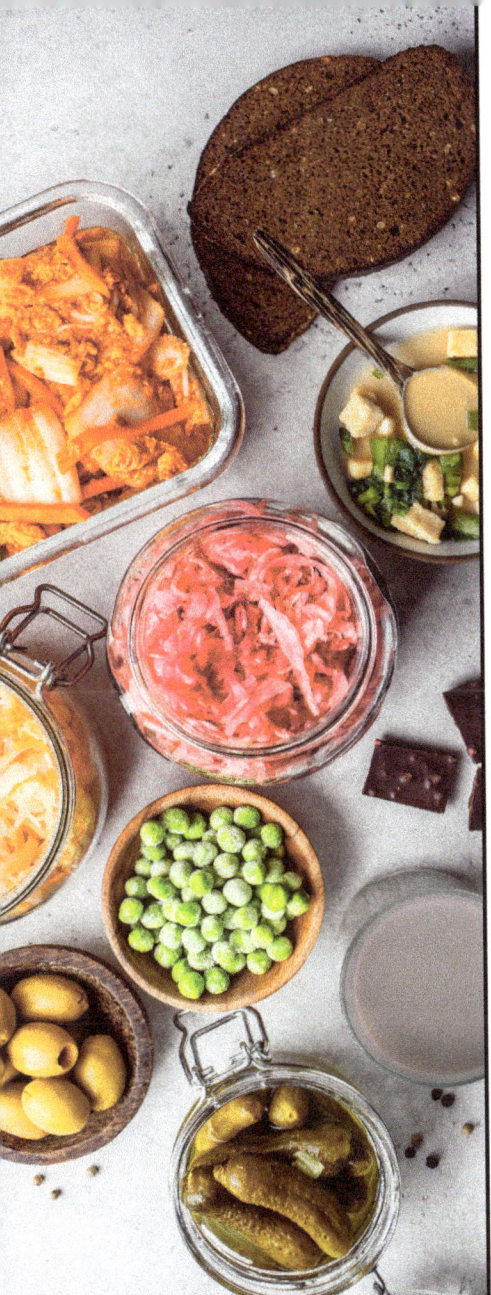

*Feed your gut flora,
fuel your health.*

- 5 -
PROBIOTIC RICH

Probiotic Rich Recipes

I talk about probiotics a lot because they're power players. These live cultures, in fermented foods, work with your gut to strengthen immune defenses, ease digestion, and even help regulate your mood (yes, really). When I travel, probiotic supplements are my first packing essential; they keep my stomach happy while I'm trying new foods abroad. But you don't need pills to get the benefits: A few daily bites of plant-based yogurt or sauerkraut do the job deliciously.

These recipes are gut gold. Foods like tempeh, miso, and coconut yogurt deliver good bacteria that balance your microbiome, help absorb nutrients, and may even curb sugar swings. Feed your microbes well, and they'll return the favor. Consider this chapter your invite to eat for two: you and your trillion microscopic allies.

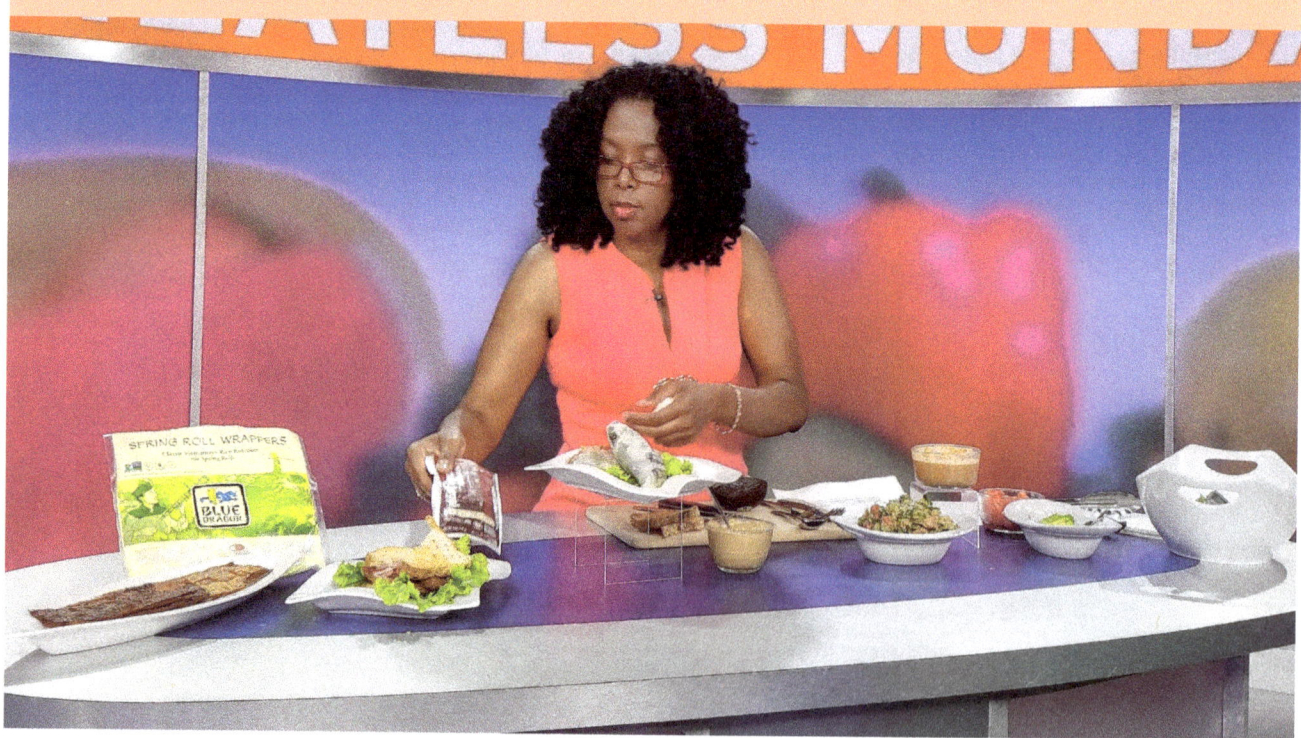

Coconut Parfait with Date-Seed Crumble

Enjoy this effortless parfait, rich in probiotics, as a quick breakfast or elegant, healthful dessert.

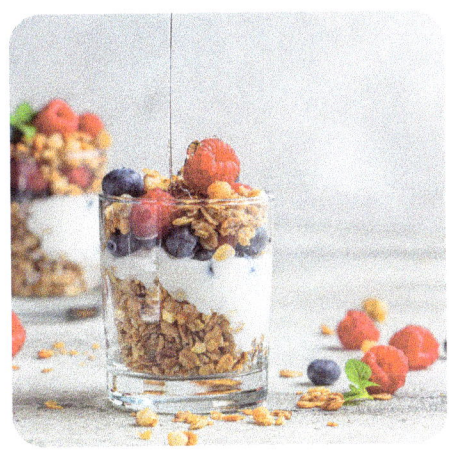

Cardamom is part of the ginger family and adds a mild warm spice flavor to sweet & savory dishes.

INGREDIENTS

½ cup   Crunchy Date-Seed Crumble
¾ cup   vanilla coconut milk yogurt (non-dairy)
½ tsp   raw agave or raw coconut nectar
¼ tsp   cardamom
¼ cup   seasonal berries, fresh

Crunchy Date-Seed Crumble

4-5   Medjool dates, pitted
3 tbsp   pumpkin seeds
1 tbsp   chia seeds (or flax seeds)
¼ tsp   cinnamon
Pinch   sea salt

1. In a food processor, pulse dates, seeds & spices until crumbly (stop before it becomes a paste).
2. For chunkier texture, hand-chop dates & mix with seeds. Keeps in the fridge for 2 weeks!

DIRECTIONS

1. Parfait layers: Yogurt → berries → crumble → repeat.
2. In a small metal bowl, mix together the coconut milk yogurt, raw agave nectar, and cardamom. Place ½ of the yogurt in the bottom of the parfait glass.
3. Place half of the the fresh berries on top of the yogurt.
4. Place half of the crumble on top of the berries.
5. Repeat with the remaining half of ingredients.

SERVINGS	TIME	LEVEL	KCAL	FIBER	CARB	FAT	PROTEIN
2	20 mins	easy	365	8g	51g	16g	12g

Waldorf Salad Remix

This is one of my absolute FAVORITE salads, such a refreshing and delicious twist on the classic.

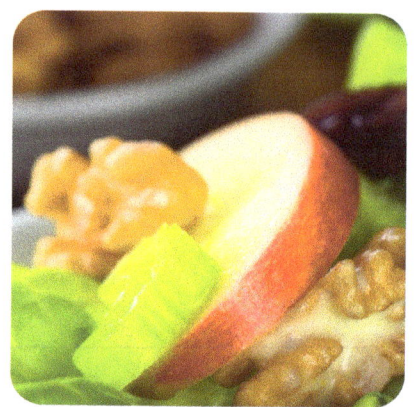

The original Waldorf salad (1893) was just apples, celery, and mayo—but we've upgraded it with dairy-free yogurt, greens, and a sweet-spiced kick!

INGREDIENTS

3/4 cup	plain, non-dairy coconut yogurt (may sub almond, oat, cashew or soy yogurt)
2 tbsp	raw agave or pure maple syrup, or coconut nectar
1 tsp	cinnamon
3	celery ribs, finely chopped
2 med	apples, chopped in to ¼ inch pieces
1 cup	red grapes, washed and removed from stem
½ cup	green grapes, washed and removed from stem
½ cup	walnuts, roughly chopped
4 cups	fresh spinach

DIRECTIONS

1. Add the yogurt, agave and cinnamon to a large bowl and whisk until well combined.
2. Add all remaining ingredients (EXCEPT the spinach) to the bowl and toss until the ingredients are well coated.
3. Serve over the fresh spinach.

SERVINGS	TIME	LEVEL	KCAL	FIBER	CARB	FAT	PROTEIN
3	20 mins	easy	342	7g	50g	14g	9g

Savory Raw Collard Green Wraps

The miso paste in this dish contains beneficial bacteria which can improve gut health and digestion. Since it is a raw recipe, the probiotics remain intact.

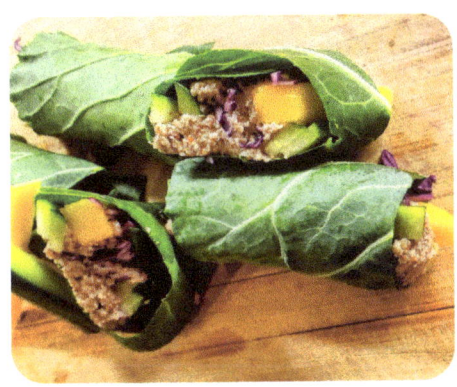

High in healthy fats and fiber from walnuts, which may improve cholesterol levels and aid in weight management.

FILLING INGREDIENTS:

1 cup	walnuts, soaked overnight or 2 hours, drained
1/4	purple cabbage, shredded (optional)
1	cucumber, diced
3 tbsp	organic white miso paste or tamari
1 clove	garlic, peeled
1/4 cup	basil leaves, fresh
1 tbsp	lemon juice
1 tbsp	apple cider vinegar
1 tsp	sea salt
1	small shallot or ½ of a red onion
dash	cracked pepper

GREENS & GARNISHES:

5	Collard green leaves, washed, stems removed, leaves cut it half along the stem line
1	cucumber, sliced into matchsticks
1	pear, sliced into thin wedges

DIRECTIONS

1. Add filling ingredients to a food processor and pulse until chunks are gone.
2. Lay collard flat with stem side up cut along both sides of the stem and remove it so it's easy to roll. If the leaves are very large cut them in half again.
3. Lay the collard leaf on a flat surface, smooth side up, and spread the walnut filling in the middle of the leaf.
4. Add 1-2 cucumber matchsticks and 1-2 pear slices, then roll the collard leaf to make a wrap.
5. Roll the leaf, starting with the base of the leaf. Secure with a toothpick.
6. Repeat with remaining filling. Serve with Sweet Chili Dipping Sauce on page 102.

SERVINGS	TIME	LEVEL	KCAL	FIBER	CARB	FAT	PROTEIN
3-4	30 mins	intermediate	284	7g	23g	20g	9g

Walnut Mushroom Cups & Miso Gravy

Why this recipe belongs here:
walnuts (prebiotics) + miso (probiotics) = a supportive microbiome blend.

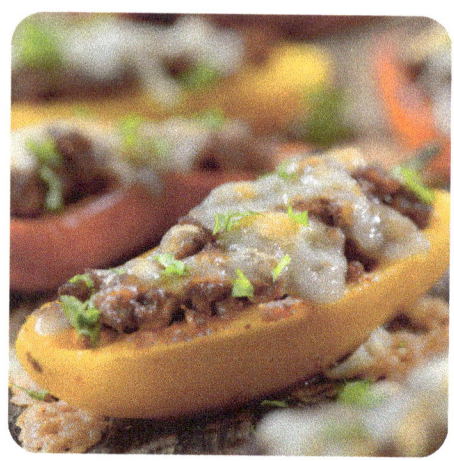

Miso gets its probiotics from fermentation. Just one tablespoon brings deep Umami flavor and supports a healthy gut with live cultures.

FILLING INGREDIENTS

1 cup	raw walnuts
1 cup	shitake mushrooms (stems removed)
1 large	shallot
¼ cup	parsley, chopped
3 tbsp	white miso paste
2 cloves	garlic
1/2 tsp	sea salt (optional)

CUP INGREDIENTS:

8	mini red/yellow bell pepper, seeded & cut in half

MISO GRAVY INGREDIENTS:

1 cup	cashews, soaked & rinsed
1.5 tbsp	fresh lemon juice
1 cup	water
½ cup	plain almond or hemp milk
3 tbsp	nutritional yeast
½ tsp	cracked pepper
2 cloves	garlic
1/4	red onion or 1 shallot
2 tbsp	red miso paste

Continued on the next page.

SERVINGS	TIME	LEVEL	KCAL	FIBER	CARB	FAT	PROTEIN
4	25 mins	Medium	531	9g	33g	37g	22g

FILLING PREPARATION:

1. Add walnuts, shallots and garlic to food processor and pulse a few times until walnuts are ground but still chucky.
2. Add mushrooms (remove stems) and all other FILLING ingredients; pulse until all ingredients are well incorporated.
3. Spoon about 1-2 tablespoons of mixture into the mini bell peppers halves and place in serving dish.

MISO GRAVY PREPARATION:

1. Add water and cashews to blender, and blend until somewhat smooth
2. Add all other ingredients to the blender and blend until smooth, creamy consistency is reached.
3. Pour gravy into serving bowl. Gravy can be slightly heated if desired.

PUTTING IT ALL TOGETHER:

Top each of the stuffed mini bell peppers with a generous dollop of the gravy. Best served at room temperature.

Serve and Enjoy!

Miso Mango Kale Salad

This is the recipe that converts kale haters to lovers! The savory dressing and the sweet mango combo is absolute perfection!

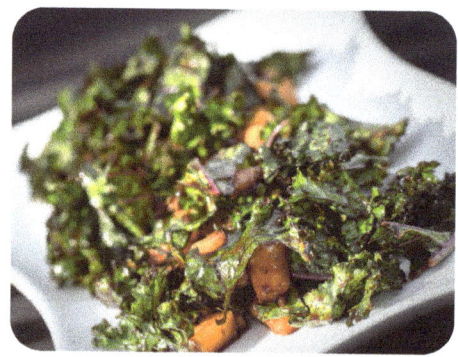

One raw cup of kale covers all your daily vitamins A, C, and K, plus a fiber boost.

INGREDIENTS

1 large	bunch curly kale, washed and torn into small pieces
2 tbsp	tamari
2 tbsp	white miso paste
2 tbsp	stone-ground mustard
2 tbsp	extra virgin olive oil (optional)
3	cloves garlic, minced
1	large lemon, juiced
1 large	ripe mango, peeled and diced into small squares (1 inch)

DIRECTIONS

1. Remove large stems from kale. Place the kale in a large bowl. Massage the kale for a minute or two to soften.
2. in a separate bowl, whisk all ingredients except kale and mango until well mixed.
3. Drizzle the over the kale and toss salad to coat all leaves with the dressing.
4. Add in the diced mango and toss well.

SERVINGS	TIME	LEVEL	KCAL	FIBER	CARB	FAT	PROTEIN
3-4	20 mins	easy	204	5g	19g	13g	6g

Sweet Potato Kale Skillet with Sauerkraut & Sour Cream

Nothing beats a savory breakfast. This dish combines tangy sauerkraut, gut-friendly sour cream, and sweet potatoes for a flavor and digestion win.

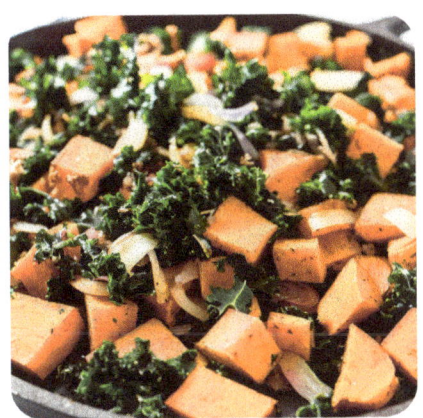

One sweet potato gives you four times your daily vitamin A, thanks to its natural beta carotene.

INGREDIENTS

2-3 med	sweet potatoes, cut into cubes (about 2.5 pounds)
1	yellow or white onion, thinly sliced
3 cups	kale, destemmed and torn into bite-sized pieces
3 cloves	garlic, minced
1 tsp	smoked paprika
1 tsp	sea salt
1/8 tsp	cracked pepper
1 tbsp	cold-pressed coconut oil (optional)
1 cup	plain or dill sauerkraut
1/2 cup	coconut sour cream (recipe on page 104)

DIRECTIONS

1. Add coconut oil to a cast iron skillet and heat. Add onions and cubed sweet potatoes and seasonings to the skillet and cook for about 10-12 minutes until onions are translucent.
2. Add kale and garlic to skillet and cook for another 3 -4 minutes.
3. Removes from heat.
4. Divide into 4-5 servings. Top with 2 tablespoons of sauerkraut and 1 tablespoon coconut sour cream.

SERVINGS	TIME	LEVEL	KCAL	FIBER	CARB	FAT	PROTEIN
4	30 mins	easy	443	7g	70g	17g	4g

Super Simple BBQ Tempeh

Tempeh is incredibly versatile and makes a great meat substitute. It shines when seasoned well!

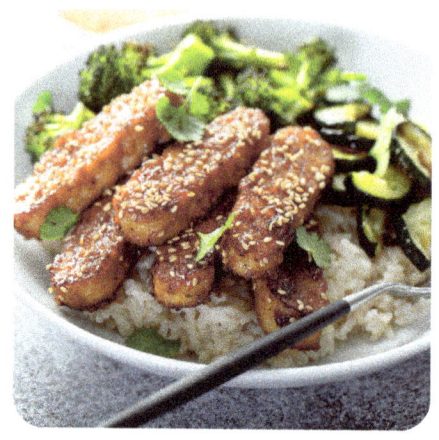

INGREDIENTS

8 oz	plain or smoky marinated tempeh
1 cup	organic BBQ sauce
3 tbsp	Dijon or brown mustard
1	red or yellow onion, sliced

Tempeh is a fermented soy product, rich in probiotics and complete protein—its natural fermentation process makes it easier to digest than plain soybeans.

DIRECTIONS

1. Slice tempeh into strips about 1 inch wide and place into a baking dish.
2. Mix Pour BBQ sauce over tempeh and mix gently to coat. Optional: cover and let marinate for 2 to 24 hours.
3. Heat skillet and add 1 tablespoon of olive oil. Add tempeh and onions to skillet and cook for about 5-7 minutes until tempeh browns. Remove from heat & serve.

SERVING SUGGESTIONS:

1. Serve on a bun with romaine lettuce, vegan mayo. For a probiotic boost, top with 2 tablespoons of sauerkraut & organic pickles. Serve with salad/coleslaw.
2. Serve with Yellow Grits with Leeks & Mushrooms (recipe on page 127), or with smoky greens (recipe on page 29) and a side of sauerkraut.

SERVINGS	TIME	LEVEL	KCAL	FIBER	CARB	FAT	PROTEIN
2-3	20 mins	easy	185	2g	14g	9g	17g

Sesame Tempeh Sliders with Sesame Slaw

Crunchy sesame slaw meets pan-seared tempeh in these hearty, flavorful sliders.

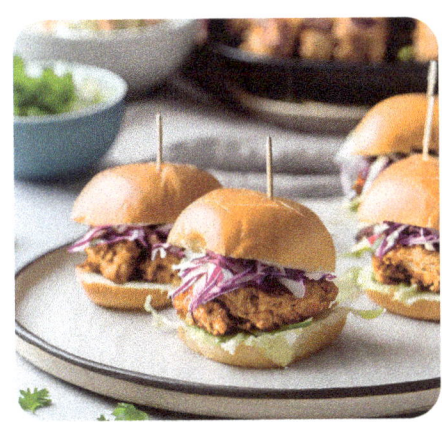

Unlike tofu, tempeh keeps the whole bean, packing more fiber and nutrients per bite.

INGREDIENTS

8 oz	marinated smoky tempeh, sliced
1/2 cup	organic hoisin sauce
2 tbsp	tamari
1 tsp	sriracha sauce
5	garlic cloves, minced
1 large	onion or shallot thinly sliced
¼ cup	cold pressed sesame oil
2 tbsp	sesame seeds
4-6 small	whole grain slider buns/rolls

SESAME SLAW

1/4 head	green cabbage, shredded
2 tbsp	vegan mayo
2 tbsp	plain brown rice vinegar
1 tbsp	sesame seeds
1 tsp	toasted sesame or olive oil
1 tsp	sriracha
1 tsp	garlic powder

DIRECTIONS

1. Heat a large skillet, add 3-4 tablespoons of water.
2. Add sliced tempeh, garlic and onions to heated skillet, let brown and caramelize on each side (about 5-7 minutes). Add more water as needed.
3. When tempeh is browned add in tamari, hoisin sauce, sriracha and sesame seeds, cook for another 5-7 minutes. Remove from heat and set aside.
4. **Slaw Prep:** Add all ingredients except cabbage to a bowl and whisk well. Pour dressing over shredded cabbage until all cabbage is coated.
5. Put slaw on bottom half of bun and top with tempeh and top half of bun.

SERVINGS	TIME	LEVEL	KCAL	FIBER	CARB	FAT	PROTEIN
2-4	30 mins	easy	358	3g	25g	24g	15g

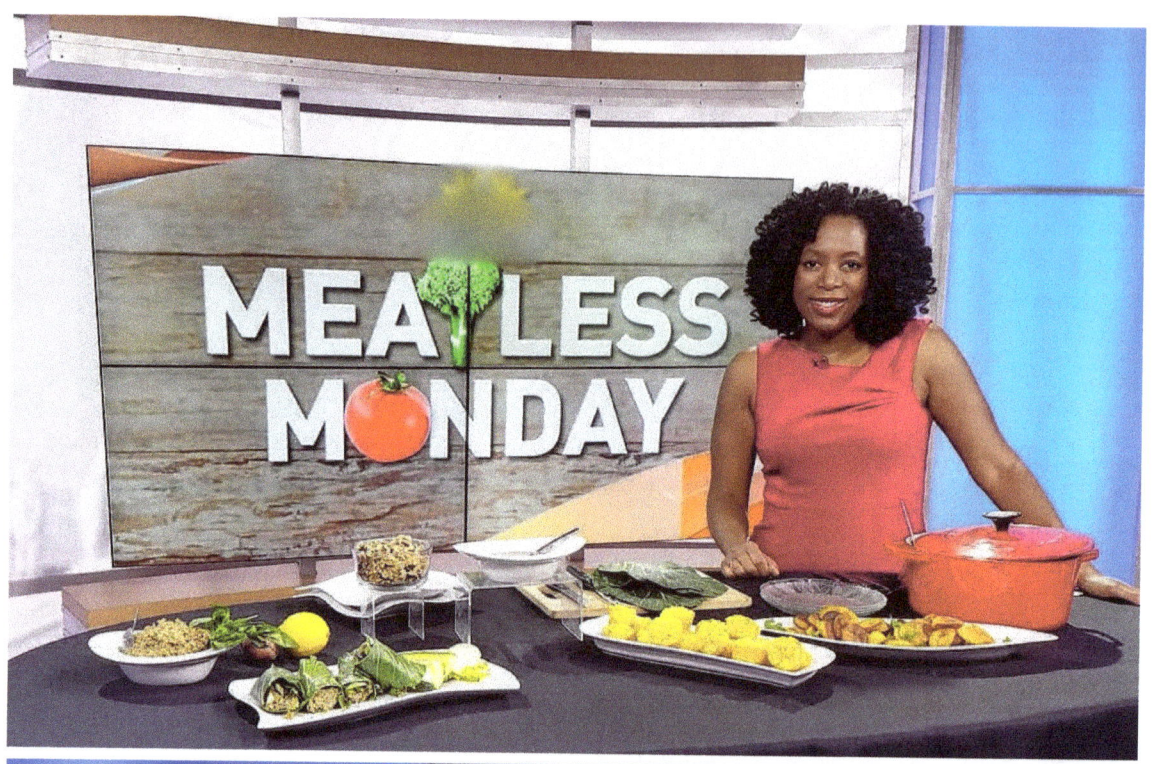

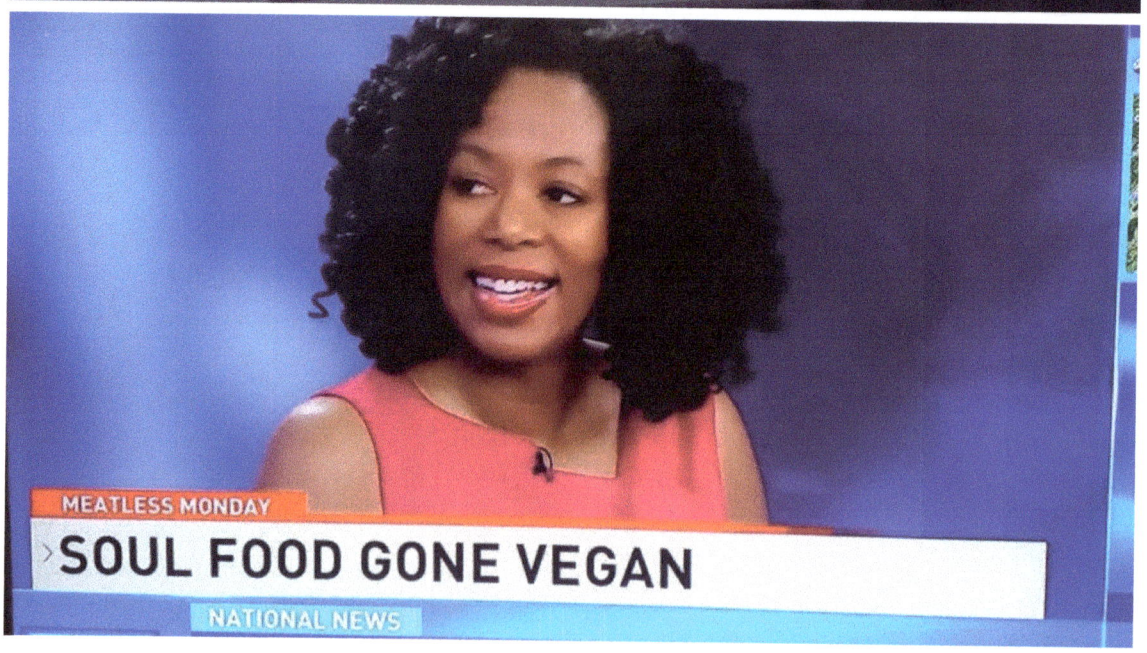

MEATLESS MONDAY

SOUL FOOD GONE VEGAN

NATIONAL NEWS

73

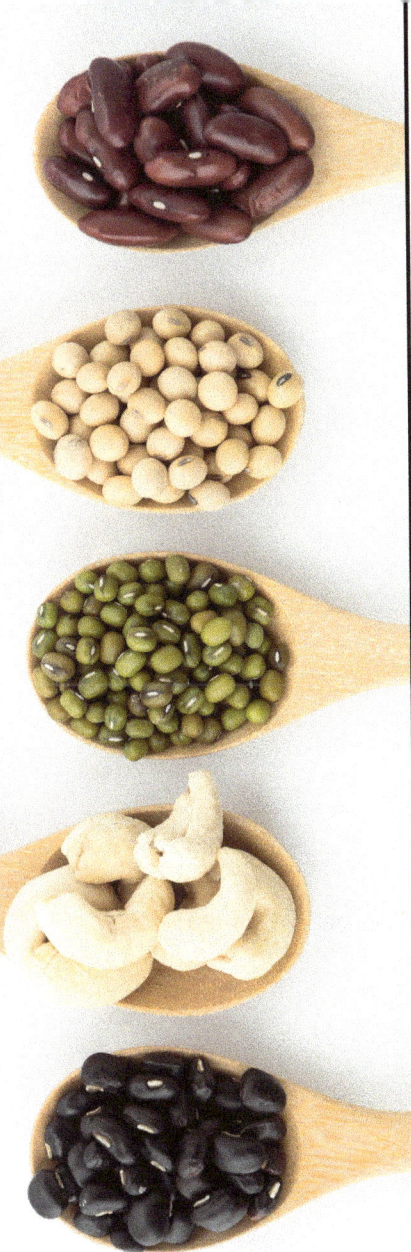

Let plants be your power.

- 6 -
PROTEIN, THE PLANT BASED WAY

Protein, the Plant Based Way

As a holistic plant-based nutritionist since 2010, I've answered one question more than any other: 'How do vegans get enough protein?' This concern comes from our cultural *protein equals meat* mindset, but here's what I've learned through years of practice and study. Every whole plant food contains protein, with certain standouts like tempeh, lentils, and quinoa offering impressive amounts. The recipes in this chapter, from smoky chili to walnut pilaf, show how satisfying and protein-rich plant based eating can be when you know how to combine and season foods effectively.

Unlike animal proteins, plants package their protein with fiber, antioxidants, and beneficial microbes. When you enjoy seitan beef and broccoli or cashew cheese pizza, you're getting complete amino acid profiles along with nutrients that support digestion and heart health. These meals prove you can meet your protein needs while nourishing your body on a deeper level. After sixteen years of vegan cooking, I can confidently say plants don't just match animal proteins they surpass them in overall nutritional value.

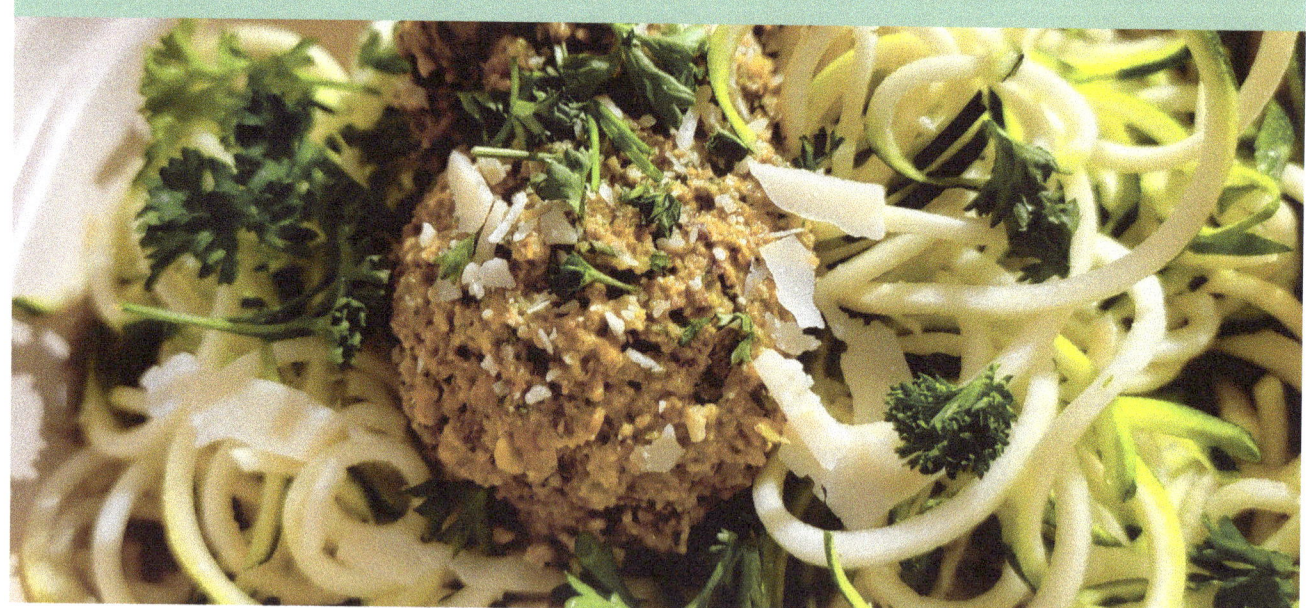

Pistachio Pesto & Zucchini Noodles

Broccoli Almond Stir Fry

Soaking almonds helps unlocks their nutrient by neutralizing enzyme inhibitors, making their protein and minerals like magnesium more absorbable. And, it gives them a tender crunch perfect for stir fries!

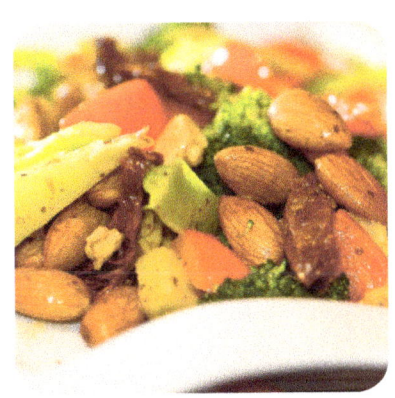

Just one ounce of almonds delivers 6g plant protein plus heart healthy fats.

INGREDIENTS

1 large	head of broccoli, cut into florets
1 large	red bell pepper, seeds removed, cut into 1-2 inch pieces
1/2 cup	raw almonds (soaked for 2 or more hours and drained)
1/4 cup	sundried tomatoes
1 tsp	dulse (seaweed)
2 tbsp	tamari
1 tsp	garlic powder
4 oz	marinated tempeh such as *Lightlife Marinated Tempeh Strips* (optional)

DIRECTIONS

1. Chop bell pepper Heat about 3-4 tablespoons of water in a wok or stainless steel pan.
2. Add tempeh and cook for 4-5 minutes to brown slightly.
3. Add broccoli, bell pepper and sundried tomatoes. Cover and let cook on medium heat for about 2 minutes, stir occasionally to prevent sticking.
4. Add all other ingredients except olive oil. Cover for another 2 minutes until broccoli is bright green and still firm.
5. Remove from heat. Serve alone or over brown rice or quinoa.

SERVINGS	TIME	LEVEL	KCAL	FIBER	CARB	FAT	PROTEIN
3	25 mins	easy	305	9g	28g	15g	18g

"Beef" & Broccoli Stir Fry

Seitan (pronounced "SAY-tan") is pure wheat gluten, with 18-24g protein per 3oz (more than some beef cuts), with zero cholesterol and a meaty texture that absorbs flavors like a sponge. So yeah, it's not gluten free, but for those who tolerate it, seitan is a high-protein option.

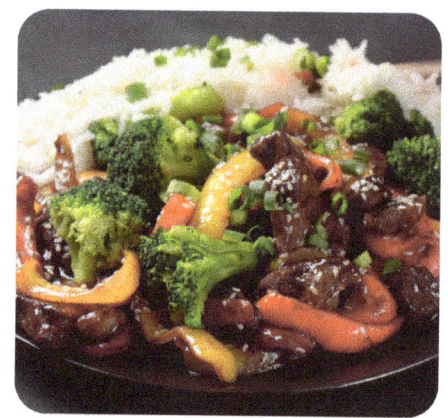

Broccoli's sulforaphane activates cellular defense pathways—researchers refer to it as a 'green shield.

INGREDIENTS

4 ounces	packaged seitan, cut into strips
1 large	head of broccoli, cut into florets
1 large	red or orange bell pepper, seeds removed, cut into 2-inch pieces
¼ cup	sundried tomatoes (rehydrated)
½ cup	hoisin sauce
1 tbsp	tamari or coconut aminos
1 clove	garlic, minced
1 tbsp	coconut oil

DIRECTIONS

1. Heat coconut oil or 4 tablespoons of water in a wok or stainless-steel pan.
2. Add seitan, hoisin and tamari and cook for 4-5 minutes to brown slightly.
3. Add broccoli, bell pepper, sundried tomatoes and garlic. Cover and let cook on medium heat for 2 minutes. Stir occasionally to prevent seitan sticking.
4. Cover for another 2 minutes or until broccoli is bright green and still firm. Remove from heat and serve. Serve over brown rice or quinoa.

SERVINGS	TIME	LEVEL	KCAL	FIBER	CARB	FAT	PROTEIN
3	20 mins	easy	177	3g	30g	5g	9g

Hearty Smokin' Chili

This plant-based chili celebrates deep, layered flavors. Blackstrap molasses brings caramel richness, while crumbled tempeh and mushrooms deliver satisfying meaty texture, no meat required.

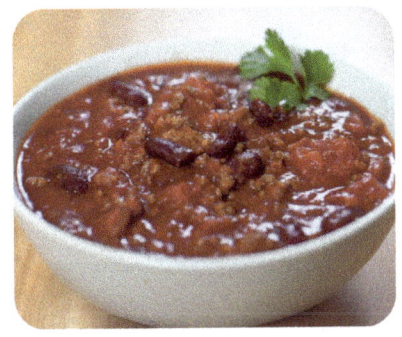

INGREDIENTS

2 cups	chili beans, soaked 8 hours or overnight and rinsed
28 oz	organic diced tomatoes, canned
2-3 tbsp	black strap molasses
6 cloves	garlic, minced
1	yellow onion, diced
1	yellow or red bell pepper, diced
½ bunch	curly parsley
¼ bunch	cilantro
4-6 oz	organic plain tempeh, crumbled
¾ cup	button mushrooms, sliced
2 tbsp	brown mustard

DRY SEASONINGS:

¼ cup	chili powder
4	bay leaves
1 tsp	paprika
1 tsp	garlic powder
1 tsp	cumin
1 tsp	oregano, dried
1 tsp	basil, dried
1 tsp	sea salt
¾ tsp	cayenne pepper
Dash	nutmeg
Dash	cinnamon
Dash	cracked pepper

Smoked paprika, (one of my favorite seasonings) gets its rich, savory flavor from peppers slowly dried over oak fires, adding a bold umami kick to vegan dishes.

Continued on the next page.

SERVINGS	TIME	LEVEL	KCAL	FIBER	CARB	FAT	PROTEIN
4-6	45 mins	Intermediate	231	5g	22g	12g	14g

Hearty Smokin' Chili - *continued*

One tablespoon of blackstrap molasses delivers 20% of your daily iron and magnesium, enriching this chili's depth.

DIRECTIONS

1. **Sauté Base Ingredients:**
   - In a large stock pot over medium heat, add coconut oil, crumbled tempeh, mushrooms, bell pepper, onions, and garlic. Cook for 5 minutes until tempeh begins to brown.
2. **Build the Chili:**
   - Add all dry seasonings, diced tomatoes, blackstrap molasses, and soaked beans. Stir well to combine, then add 6 cups water and bring to a boil.
3. **Simmer:**
   - Reduce heat to low, cover, and simmer for 30 minutes.
4. **Finish:**
   - Stir in cilantro and parsley. Continue cooking uncovered for 20-30 more minutes until beans are tender, stirring occasionally.
   - Add water as needed to prevent sticking and according to thickness preference.
   - Adjust seasonings to taste
   - Remove bay leaves before serving

Note: If using canned beans, reduce cooking time by 30 minutes and use half as much water.

Sprouted Cranberry Quinoa

Sprouted quinoa is simply quinoa that's been soaked and rinsed until it begins to germinate, making it easier to digest and unlocking more of its natural nutrients. You can find packaged sprouted quinoa at most health food stores.

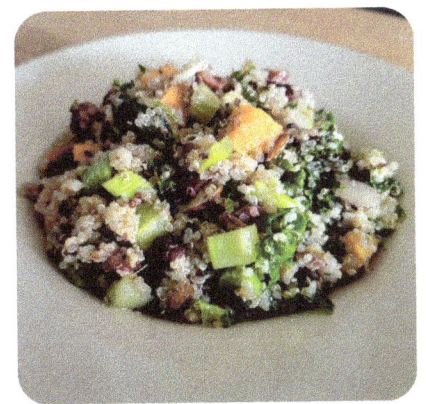

Sunflower seeds' healthy fats help your body absorb kale's iron, while their vitamin E protects cells.

INGREDIENTS

3 cups	sprouted quinoa, prepared
1 cup	dried organic cranberries
1.5 cup	diced sweet potatoes, roasted
1 cup	parsley, chopped
1/2 cup	green onions (scallions)
¼ cup	raw sunflower seeds
3 stalks	chopped celery
6 tbsp	organic red wine vinegar
2 tbsp	fresh lemon juice
2 tsp	extra virgin olive oil
1 tsp	sea salt or to taste
3 cups	curly kale, torn into bite size pieces

DIRECTIONS

1. Cook sprouted quinoa per label instructions–in broth instead of water for increased flavor.
2. Spread diced sweet potatoes on a parchment-lined baking sheet. Roast at 400°F for 25 minutes, flipping once halfway, until tender and caramelized at the edges.
3. Once sweet potatoes are done, Put them in large mixing bowl along with the cooked quinoa; set aside.
4. In a separate bowl mix red wine vinegar, lemon juice, olive oil, sea salt, & parsley with a whisk.
5. Tear kale and mix with quinoa/sweet potatoes. Pour dressing over mixture and mix until well coated.
6. Mix in the the cranberries, raisins, celery, green onions, and sunflower seeds. Chill.

SERVINGS	TIME	LEVEL	KCAL	FIBER	CARB	FAT	PROTEIN
4-6	30 mins	easy	464	10g	77g	10g	10g

Quick & Easy Black Bean Pita

Whip up a batch of these protein-packed pockets on Sunday; stuff them with spiced beans, diced veggies, and avocado for grab-and-go lunches all week.

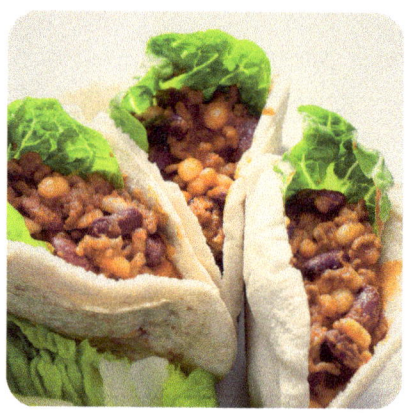

Black beans and hemp seeds together make a complete protein—all nine essential amino acids in one easy meal.

INGREDIENTS

1 cup	cooked black beans
1/2	avocado, diced
1 small	tomato, diced
1 small	tomatillo, diced
1/2	yellow bell pepper, seeded & diced
1/2 tsp	cumin
1/2 tsp	chili powder
1/2 tsp	cayenne pepper
1/2 tsp	sea salt
2-3	romaine lettuce leaves
1-2	whole gain or gluten-free pita pockets, cut in half
1 tsp	hempseeds

DIRECTIONS

1. Heat beans in a sauce pan for 4-6. While cooking, mash beans with back of spoon.
2. Add cumin, chili powder, seal salt and cayenne to the beans and mix well.
3. In a separate bowl, mix diced tomato, tomatillo, bell pepper and avocado.
4. Add lettuce to pita, then add a couple of spoons of beans and top with 3-4 tablespoons of the tomato, tomatillo mixture, then sprinle with hemp seeds for more protein.

Serving option: serve on a bed of lettuce, without pita.

SERVINGS	TIME	LEVEL	KCAL	FIBER	CARB	FAT	PROTEIN
3	20 mins	easy	311	13g	50g	8g	14g

Raw Veggie Max Pizza

This vibrant, no-bake pizza layers a almond crust, creamy cashew cheese, and a rainbow of fresh veggies into one nutrient-dense meal; no oven required.

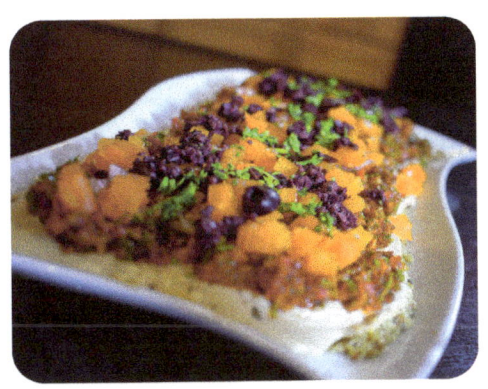

For a nut free alternative, sunflower seeds can be substituted for the almonds & tahini for the cashews.

TOPPINGS:

¾ cup	cherry tomatoes, diced
½ cup	sundried tomatoes, chopped
¾ cup	yellow or orange bell peppers, diced
½ cup	Kalamata olives, diced
½	red onion, chopped
¾ cup	fresh parsley, chopped
1 tbsp	oregano
1 tsp	tamari
½ tsp	sea salt
½ tsp	fresh lemon juice
dash	cracked pepper, sprinkle on top

CASHEW CHEESE INGREDIENTS:

1 cup	raw cashews, soaked for 2 - 24 hours, drained
1	lemon, juiced
2 tbsp	nutritional yeast
1 tbsp	olive oil
½ -1 tsp	sea salt
3 cloves	garlic
1 tbsp	tamari
¼ cup	purified water

CRUST INGREDIENTS:

1 cup	raw almonds, soaked 2-24 hours, drained
1/2 cup	fresh basil
1/2 tsp	sea salt
1 clove	garlic

Continued on next page.

SERVINGS	TIME	LEVEL	KCAL	FIBER	CARB	FAT	PROTEIN
4	30 mins	Advanced	595	9g	37g	43g	23g

CRUST DIRECTIONS:
1. Add all ingredients to a food processor and pulse until nuts are very finely chopped and able to be molded into a dish.
2. Scoop into the serving dish (i.e., large plate, pie dish, individual ramekins, etc.).
3. Press into serving dish to make a tight thin crust, closing all gaps.

CASHEW CHEESE DIRECTIONS:
1. Blend all ingredients together in a high speed blender until smooth. Add enough water to mixture to keep blender moving.
2. Mixture should be thick and slightly pourable. Scoop out with a spatula and spread a thick layer gently onto nut crust.
3. Use immediately or refrigerate for later use—cheese will thicken after chilled for 3 or more hours.

TOPPINGS DIRECTIONS:
1. Add cherry tomatoes sundried tomatoes to a food processor and pulse until coarsely chopped. Set aside.
2. Add onions, parsley, lemon juice and tamari to a food processor and pulse until diced.
3. Chop olives and bell pepper separately and set aside (optional – you can mix these with the other veggies if desired)
4. Add veggies except olives and bell peppers to the tomato sauce and add oregano, lemon juice and tamari. Mix all veggies together until well mixed.
5. Set aside until ready to place on pizza.

PUTTING IT ALL TOGETHER:
1. Scoop or pour cheese sauce gently onto nut crust and spread a thick even layer.
2. Add chopped vegetable toppings on top of cheese, evenly to cover. Some cheese should be visible around the edges.
3. Spoon a few dollops of cashew cheese on top and top with cracked pepper.
4. Serve immediately.

Serving Suggestion: Serve at room temperature with a mixed green salad.

Cholesterol Free Tempeh Sloppy Joes

Only animal products contain dietary cholesterol. Tempeh, made from soybeans, provides complete protein without cholesterol, and its fermentation adds gut-friendly benefits too!

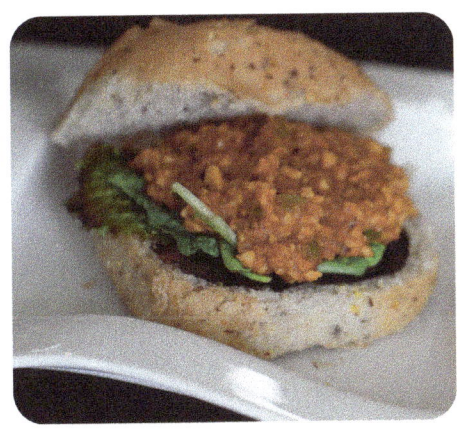

This recipe swaps beef for tempeh, trading saturated fat for fiber and probiotics.

INGREDIENTS

8 oz	plain organic tempeh, crumbled
16 oz	organic barbeque sauce
2 tbsp	vegan Worcestershire sauce
1 large	yellow onion, finely diced
1	green pepper, very finely diced
1	carrot, peeled and finely shredded
4	cloves garlic, minced
2 tbsp	stone ground brown mustard
2 tbsp	cold pressed coconut oil
1 tbsp	organic tomato paste
½ tsp	cracked pepper
4	whole grain buns

DIRECTIONS

1. Heat a large skillet, add 3-4 tablespoons of water.
2. Add crumbled tempeh, green peppers, garlic and onions to heated skillet, let brown and caramelize, add more water as needed (about 5-7 minutes).
3. After about 6 minutes when tempeh is almost done add 2 tablespoons of coconut oil to help brown, add carrots, cook for another 3 minutes.
4. Add barbeque sauce and mustard and let simmer for about 5 minutes.
5. Add shredded lettuce on bottom of bun, spoon on tempeh and add top bun.

SERVINGS	TIME	LEVEL	KCAL	FIBER	CARB	FAT	PROTEIN
3	20 mins	easy	750	10g	131g	17g	26g

Tuscan White Bean Penne

Garlic-infused cannellini beans cling to nutty brown rice pasta, with pops of color from spinach and sundried tomatoes—simple, rustic, and satisfying.

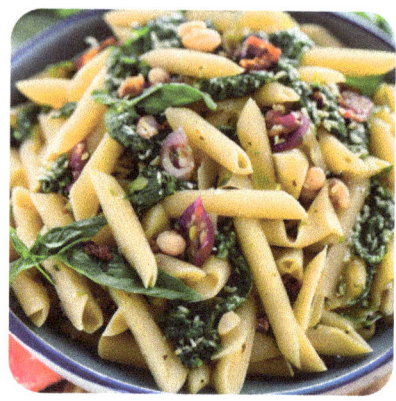

High protein gluten free pasta options include chickpea, quinoa, lentil or mung bean pastas.

INGREDIENTS

10 -12 oz	penne brown rice pasta or bowtie noodles
1 cup	cannellini beans, cooked & drained; or 15 oz canned cannellini beans, drained
4	cloves garlic, minced
1/2 cup	sundried tomatoes, chopped
2 cups	baby spinach
1	red onion, thinly sliced
3 tbsp	nutritional yeast
1 tbsp	parsley or 1/4 cup fresh parsley
1 tbsp	olive oil (optional)
1 tsp	paprika
½ tsp	sea salt, cracked pepper & cayenne pepper

DIRECTIONS

1. Prepare pasta as directed on box. Cook pasta until it is al dente, about 8 min; it will continue cooking even after it is removed from the water.
2. In a stainless steel pan/pot add garlic, onions, sundried tomatoes and 2 tablespoons of water, over medium heat. Sauté for about 1 minute.
3. Add beans and stir until beans are heated through.
4. Add cooked pasta, parsley and spinach to pan and stir until all ingredients are mixed well and spinach begins to wilt. Add 3 tbsp of water if needed.
5. Add nutritional yeast, sea salt, cracked pepper, cayenne and olive oil, and mix well. Adjust seasonings to your preference.

SERVINGS	TIME	LEVEL	KCAL	FIBER	CARB	FAT	PROTEIN
3	20 mins	easy	340	12g	55g	6g	18g

Wild Rice Pilaf with Pine Nuts

Wild Rice is one of the few grains that has all 9 essential amino acids, especially when paired with lysine-rich pine nuts, making this pilaf a complete protein powerhouse.

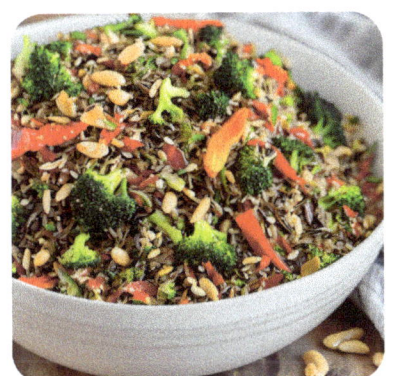

I love the nutty flavor and firm texture of wild rice. It's also lower in carbs than most grains—about 32g net carbs per cooked cup (vs. 45g in brown rice), with more protein and fiber to balance it.

INGREDIENTS

1 cup	wild rice, uncooked
3	green onions, thinly sliced
1/2	red bell pepper, diced
1/2 cup	broccoli, finely chopped
½ cup	organic corn
¼ cup	sundried tomatoes (rehydrated or packed in oil), chopped
¼ cup	pine nuts
2	garlic cloves, minced
3 tbsp	chickpea or soy miso or sub with 5 tbsp tamari
1 5-inch	strip of kombu seaweed
1 tbsp	extra-virgin olive oil (optional)
½ bunch	parsley
½ tsp	sea salt (or to taste)
¼ tsp	cracked pepper

DIRECTIONS

1. Add the kombu and miso to 3 cups of water in a medium sauce pan.
2. Bring the water to a boil.
3. Stir in one cup of wild rice, and bring rice and water to boil. Reduce heat to low and let simmer, covered.
4. Cook for about 45 minutes until kernels and rice is tender but firm. Remove from heat and drain any remaining water. Remove kombu.
5. Add in all remaining ingredients to the wild rice and mix well and cover pot to allow other ingredients to warm slightly for about 5 minutes. Serve warm.

SERVINGS	TIME	LEVEL	KCAL	FIBER	CARB	FAT	PROTEIN
2-3	65 mins	easy	409	7g	58g	15g	18g

One-Pan Garlic Miso Greens & Beans

I love simple, flavorful dishes that can be made in under 20 minutes. The tangy glaze, with bright pops of lemon and miso bring this dish alive, because nutrient dense should never mean boring. It's flexible, so swap in any greens or beans you love.

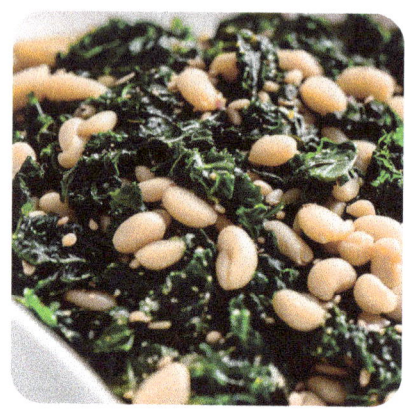

Greens like kale & beans like cannellini are rich in calcium and magnesium, but their absorption is boosted when paired with vitamin C (like lemon juice) and slowed by excess salt or caffeine.

INGREDIENTS

2 cups	cooked cannellini beans or 16-ounce canned beans
1 bunch	green curly kale, thick stems removed, chopped or torn into medium pieces
5	cloves cloves, minced
2 tbsp	chickpea or soy white miso paste
1 tbsp	red wine vinegar
1 tsp	sweet paprika or smoked paprika
1 tsp	sea salt (or to taste)
½ tsp	cayenne pepper or red pepper flakes
1 tsp	lemon juice
1 tbsp	cold-pressed coconut oil (optional)

DIRECTIONS

1. Add minced garlic to pan and sauté with water or a little oil.
2. Add in miso and ½ cup of water and stir until miso paste dissolves.
3. Add greens to pan and let cook for 2-3 minutes.
4. Add beans, sea salt, paprika, cayenne pepper and red wine vinegar; mix well.
5. Cook until greens are wilted and beans are heated through and water has cooked out.
6. Remove from heat and squeeze lemon juice on top & stir. Serve warm.

SERVINGS	TIME	LEVEL	KCAL	FIBER	CARB	FAT	PROTEIN
3	30 mins	easy	294	12g	45g	7g	16g

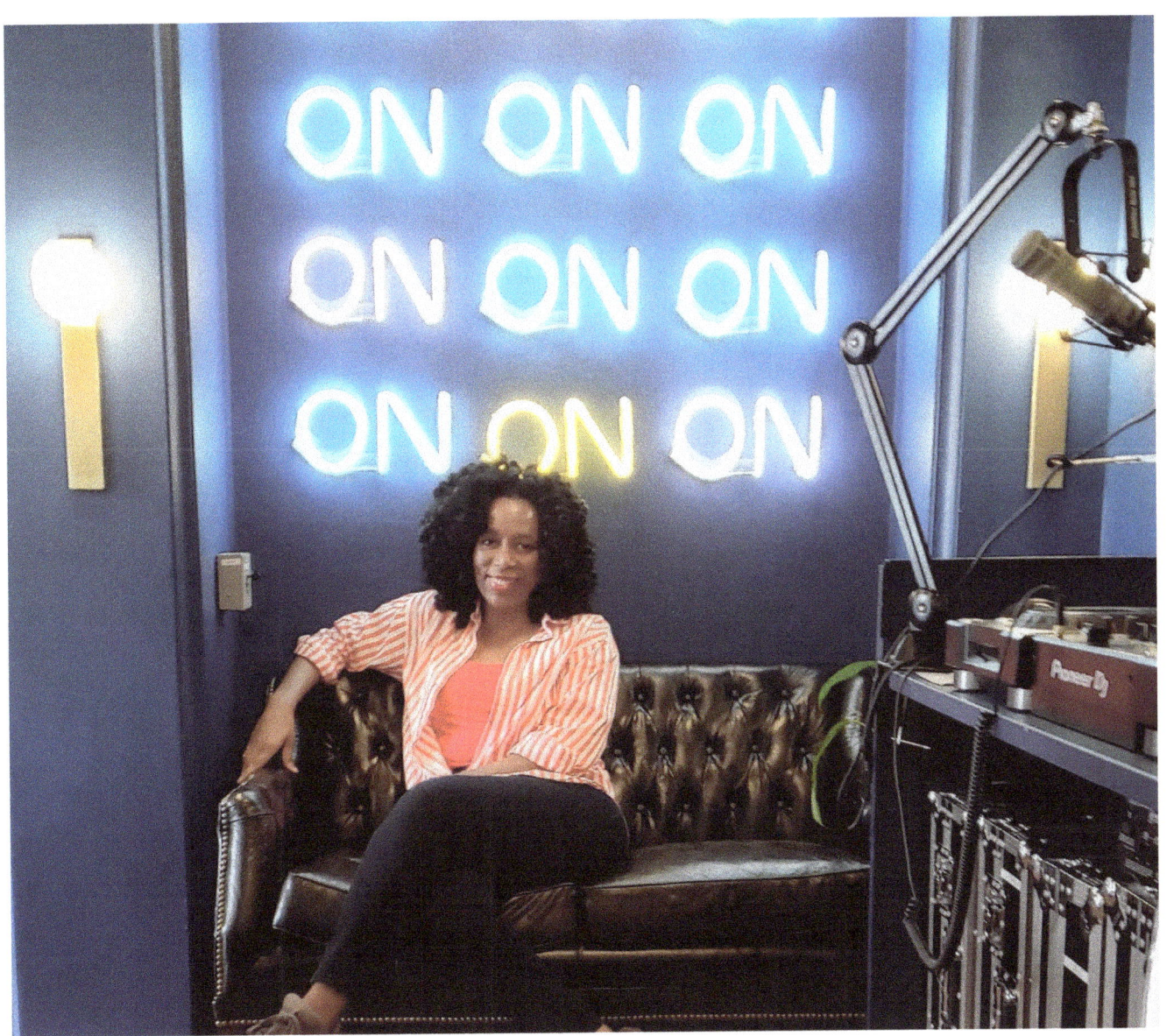

Going on air in...

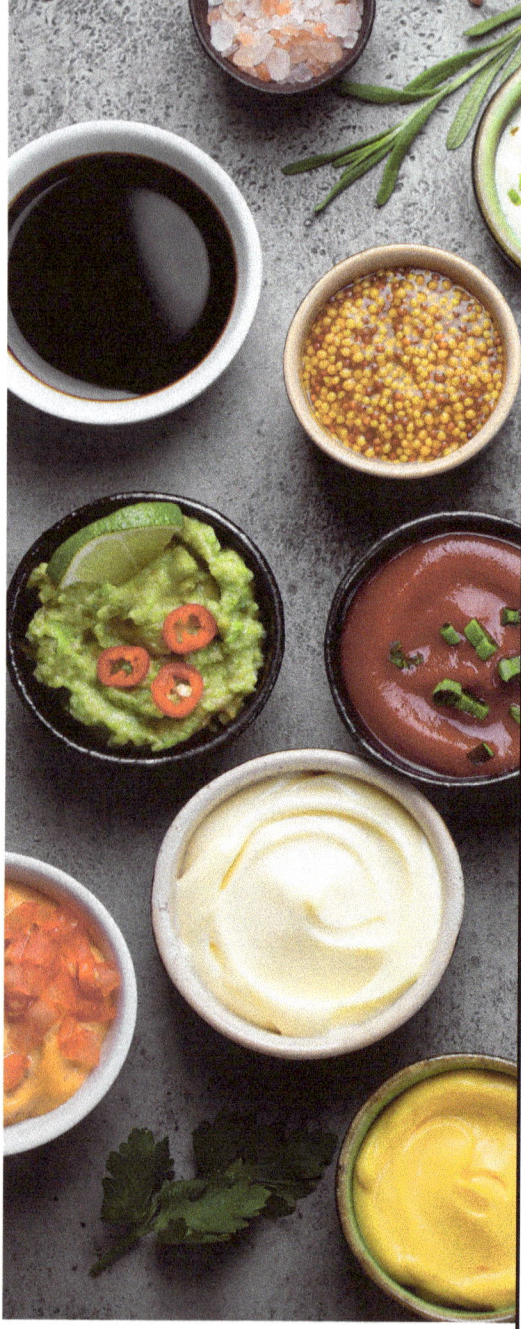

Dress boldly. Dip deeply.

Dressings, Dips & Cheeses

I'm a self-proclaimed dip enthusiast. There's something magical about how a rich creamy dip or zesty salsa can transform raw veggies and simple meals into something exceptional. These recipes celebrate how plant-based dips and dressings bring big flavor while bringing nutrients like healthy fats from nuts, antioxidants from herbs, and gut-friendly probiotics from fermented ingredients.

A great dressing doesn't just complement a dish, it defines it. Drizzle ginger tahini dressing over steamed greens for an iron-boosting vitamin C kick, or toss grains in herbed hemp seed dressing for omega-3s and protein. The best part? These vegan versions come together in minutes with just a blender or food processor, and whole food ingredients. Meal prep tip: Batch dressings or dips on Sunday; they often improve after a day as flavors meld, making weeknight meals easy.

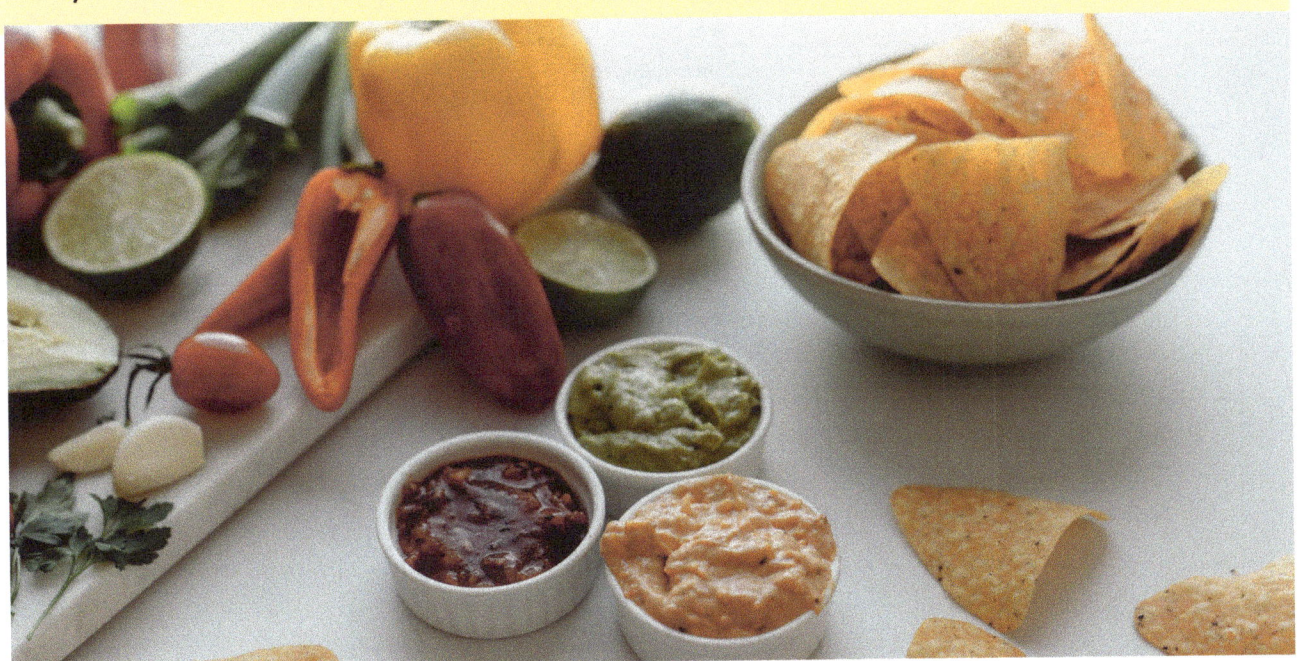

Give me ALL of the dips!

Creamy Kale and Artichoke Dip

This has all of the creamy, garlicky joy of the original, with an upgrade of sea minerals and plant protein.

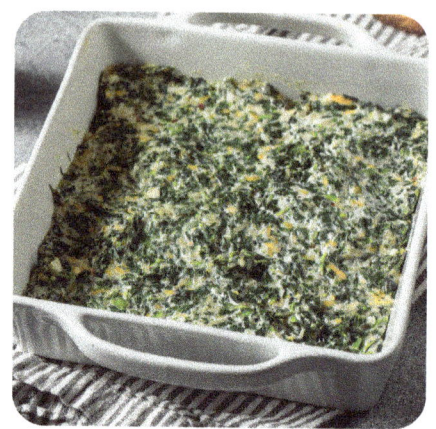

Soaked cashews blend into velvety richness, while kale and artichokes add iron and gut-friendly fiber.

INGREDIENTS

1 bunch	kale
20 oz	artichoke hearts, diced
1.5 cups	cashews, soaked 2 or more hours
½-¾ cups	water
1	lemon, juiced
4-5	cloves garlic, minced
5 tbsp	nutritional yeast
1 tsp	sea salt, or to taste
1 tsp	dulse flakes (seaweed)
1/2 tsp	cayenne pepper or to taste
½ cup	brown rice bread crumbs (optional)

DIRECTIONS

1. Blend all ingredients until smooth, except kale and artichokes. Add water as needed to keep mixture moving.
2. Remove stems from kale leaves and tear into bit size pieces. Massage kale for 1-2 minutes, until soft.
3. Mix diced artichokes and kale together in a bowl. Pour cashew mixture over kale and artichokes. Mix well.
4. Pour into baking dish. Top with gluten free bread crumbs if desired.
5. Bake in oven at 375F for 25 minutes. Remove from oven, stir &serve.

SERVINGS	TIME	LEVEL	KCAL	FIBER	CARB	FAT	PROTEIN
4	40 mins	intermediate	586	10g	39g	38g	28g

5-Minute Cashew Dip

Mild, creamy, and endlessly adaptable—thin with water for a dressing, or keep it thicker as a veggie dip.

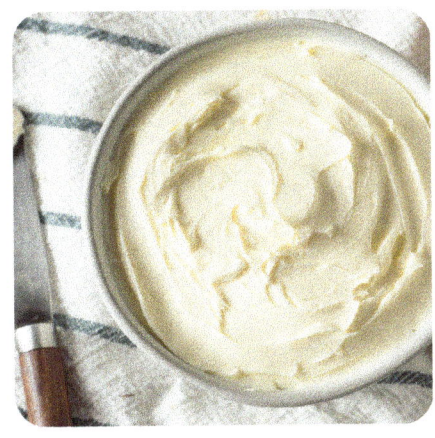

Soaked cashews blend into velvety textures because their healthy fats emulsify effortlessly, while their natural starches thicken without gums or dairy.

INGREDIENTS

1 cup	raw cashews (soaked 2 hours or more and drained)
1/2	yellow bell pepper, seeded
1 tbsp	lemon juice
1 tsp	dill, dried (3 tablespoons fresh dill)
1 clove	garlic
½-1 tsp	sea salt
½ tsp	paprika
⅓ cup	water

DIRECTIONS

1. Add all dip ingredients to a blender.
2. Blend until smooth. Adjust water as desired for thinner dressing or less for a thicker dip.

SERVINGS	TIME	LEVEL	KCAL	FIBER	CARB	FAT	PROTEIN
4	20 mins	easy	328	3g	21g	25g	11g

Zesty Tomatillo Hummus (Raw)

Sprouting chickpeas for 24–48 hours increases their protein bioavailability and reduces phytic acid, making their iron and zinc easier to absorb, while adding a fresh, slightly nutty flavor.

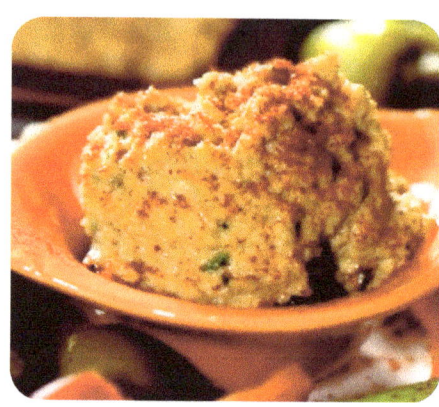

After soaking, let sit on countertop and rinse sprouts every 12 hours to keep them fresh. The tiny tails means their sprouting with big nutrition!

INGREDIENTS

2.5 cups	dried chickpeas, soak for 24 hours; drain & let sit for 24 hours to sprout, rinsing every 12 hrs
3 tbsp	tahini (sesame seed paste)
2 tbsp	tamari
2 tbsp	olive oil
1	lemon, juiced
4 cloves	garlic
3	sundried tomatoes, chopped
1	tomatillo, or sub with 1 small green tomato
1/2	bunch parsley (can substitute cilantro)
1 tsp	cumin
1 tsp	sea salt
1/2-1 tsp	chili powder
1/2-1 tsp	cayenne
2-4 tbsp	water

DIRECTIONS

1. Drain & rinse soaked chickpeas. Add chickpeas and garlic to a food processor; pulse until chickpeas are chopped.
2. Add all other ingredients to food processor except water and olive oil.
3. Process until ingredients are well incorporated, add olive oil while processing. Add water until desired thickness/looseness is achieved.
4. Taste and adjust seasonings as needed. Serve immediately or refrigerate.
5. Garnish with chopped tomatoes & serve with fresh vegetables or crackers.

SERVINGS	TIME	LEVEL	KCAL	FIBER	CARB	FAT	PROTEIN
4	20 mins	intermediate	281	8g	28g	16g	10g

Tangy Tomatillo Salsa

I love this tangy salsa and use it as an alternative to a traditional salsa whenever I want to add more zing. The green tomatillos bring a citrusy punch of flavor.

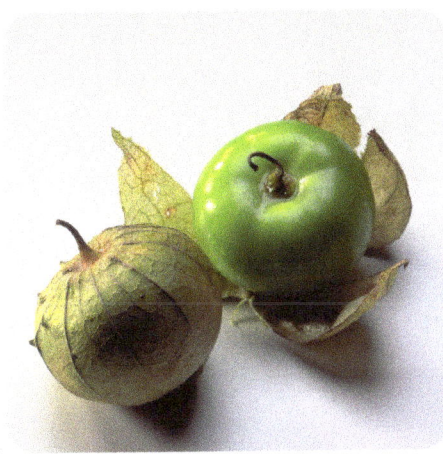

Tomatillos aren't just unripe tomatoes, they're a separate fruit high in vitamin C and a signature tartness that defines salsa verde.

INGREDIENTS

3 med	tomatillos
3 med	vine-ripened tomatoes
7 cloves	garlic
½ bunch	fresh cilantro (1 cup chopped)
1 small	jalapeno, seeded (for additional heat, include the seeds)
1 tsp	cumin
1 tsp	sea salt
½ tsp	cayenne (or to taste)

DIRECTIONS

1. Add all ingredients to a food processor and pulse until ingredients are mixed but still chunky.
2. Serve immediately or cover and let chill for 1 hour or more.

SERVINGS	TIME	LEVEL	KCAL	FIBER	CARB	FAT	PROTEIN
3	20 mins	easy	50	2g	10g	1g	2g

Creamy Poppy Seed Dressing

I'm not a fan of most bottled dressings—too many unhealthy additives—*buuuut* I also don't want to spend ages making something from scratch. Enter THIS easy dressing: no blender needed, just a whisk and gut-friendly ingredients!

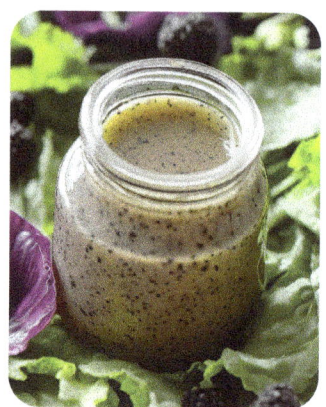

Apple cider vinegar and coconut yogurt team up for probiotics + digestion support, while poppy seeds add bone-strengthening minerals like calcium & manganese.

INGREDIENTS

½ cup	plain coconut yogurt (non-dairy)
⅓ cup	organic apple cider vinegar
2 tbsp	extra virgin olive oil (optional)
2 tbsp	pure maple syrup
1.5 tbsp	brown mustard
1 tsp	lemon juice
1 small	shallot, minced
1 tbsp	poppy seeds
1 tsp	sea salt

DIRECTIONS

1. Whisk all ingredients in a bowl until well incorporated OR pulse in food processor or blender until well mixed.
2. Makes approximately 1 cup of dressing.
3. Store refrigerated for 5 days.

SERVINGS	TIME	LEVEL	KCAL	FIBER	CARB	FAT	PROTEIN
6-10	20 mins	easy	87	1g	8g	6g	1g

Herbed Hemp Seed Dressing

I always keep hemp seeds around, they're an easy, complete protein with omega-3s and magnesium, and they actually taste good (mild and nutty).

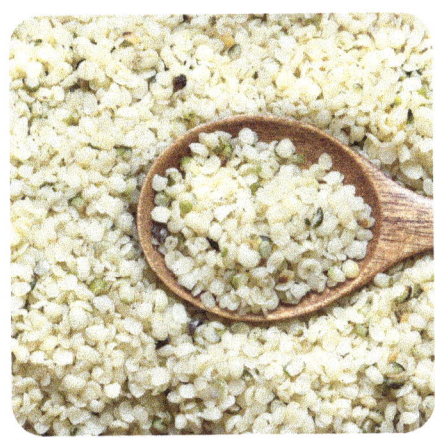

A sprinkle of hemp seeds provides stress-soothing magnesium and immune-supporting zinc, easy nutrition.

INGREDIENTS

1/2 cup	raw hemp seeds
1/2 cup	water
1/2	yellow bell pepper, seeded
2 cloves	garlic
1/4 cup	fresh basil
1/4 cup	fresh parsley
1 tbsp	apple cider vinegar
1 tbsp	brown mustard
2 tsp	nutritional yeast
3/4 tsp	sea salt

DIRECTIONS

1. Place all ingredients into a blender.
2. Blend together until smooth. Add more water for thinner dressing.
3. Serve immediately or store refrigerated for 5-7 days.

Alternative method to avoid a green colored dressing. Blend all ingredients until smooth, except basil and parsley. Finely chop basil and parsley. Pour dressing into a bowl. Add chopped basil and parsley and mix with a whisk.

SERVINGS	TIME	LEVEL	KCAL	FIBER	CARB	FAT	PROTEIN
6	20 mins	easy	134	2g	5g	10g	9g

Ginger Tahini Dressing

Creamy tahini meets zesty ginger and lemon for a refreshing dressing that cuts through hearty greens like cabbage. Try it with shredded cabbage and diced apples for a crisp, bright combo that never fails.

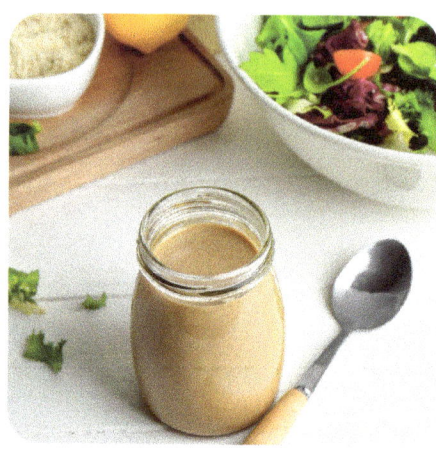

Tahini's healthy fats helps absorption of fat-soluble vitamins in cabbage (like vitamin K), while ginger aids digestion.

INGREDIENTS

4 tbsp	tahini
1 med	Roma tomato
2 inches	fresh ginger, cut in ½ inch pieces
3 tbsp	gluten-free tamari
1 tbsp	extra-virgin olive oil
1 tbsp	hempseed or flaxseed oil
2 tbsp	fresh lemon juice
4	cloves garlic
½ tsp	cumin
¼ tsp	smoked paprika

DIRECTIONS

1. Add all dressing ingredients to a food processor or blender and blend until smooth.
2. Sprinkle with additional paprika to garnish.
3. Serve immediately or cover and refrigerate. Makes about 1 cup of dressing.

SERVINGS	TIME	LEVEL	KCAL	FIBER	CARB	FAT	PROTEIN
4-6	15 mins	easy	171	3g	7g	15g	5g

Herbed Sweet Mustard Dressing & Marinade

Bright lemon, peppermint, and cilantro elevate this sweet-shallot mustard blend into a multitasker. Drizzle it on salads or marinate tofu for a few hours before cooking.

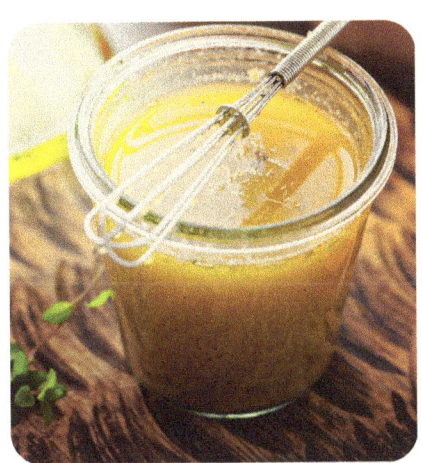

Grade B (Dark Amber) maple syrup has a more complex flavor and trace minerals than light grades.

INGREDIENTS

¼ cup	raw coconut nectar or grade B (dark) maple syrup
¼ cup	extra virgin olive oil
2-3 tbsp	stone ground brown mustard or Dijon mustard
1 small	shallot, peeled roughly chopped
1 tbsp	lemon juice
¼ cup	fresh cilantro
¼ cup	fresh peppermint
¼ tsp	sea salt
¼ tsp	paprika

DIRECTIONS

1. Add all dressing ingredients to a food processor or blender and blend until smooth.
2. Serve immediately or cover and refrigerate. Makes about 1 cup of dressing.
3. For a thicker or oil free dressing substitute the olive oil with plain, unsweetened vegan yogurt.

SERVINGS	TIME	LEVEL	KCAL	FIBER	CARB	FAT	PROTEIN
4-6	20 mins	easy	151	1g	15g	10g	1g

Lemon Garlic Salad Dressing

People absolutely love this dressing—and for good reason. Zesty lemon, punchy garlic, and nutty flax oil come together in a bright blend that upgrades any salad.

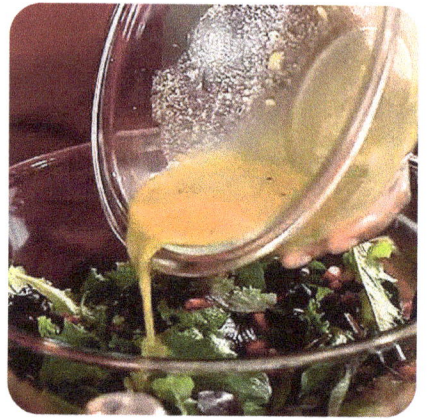

Flaxseed oil's omega-3s are heat-sensitive, but in raw dressings like this, they stay intact to support heart and brain health.

INGREDIENTS

1	lemon, juiced (or 4 tbsp)
2	cloves garlic, minced
2 tbsp	flax seed oil or hemp oil (always keep refrigerated)
2 tbsp	cold pressed olive oil
1 tbsp	nutritional yeast
1 tbsp	apple cider vinegar
1/4 tsp	cracked pepper or to taste
Dash of	sea salt (optional) or to taste
2 tbsp	water

DIRECTIONS

1. Whisk all ingredients together until well blended.
2. Use immediately or store in refrigerator for 4-5 days. A little goes a long way. Use 1 tablespoon to marinate a small to medium salad or more for a larger salad.

SERVINGS	TIME	LEVEL	KCAL	FIBER	CARB	FAT	PROTEIN
4-8	15 mins	easy	138	2g	5g	13g	3g

Fresh Cranberry Mint Vinaigrette with Arugula Walnut Salad

Tart cranberries, bright citrus, and cool mint blend into a holiday-worthy dressing, but can be enjoyed anytime!

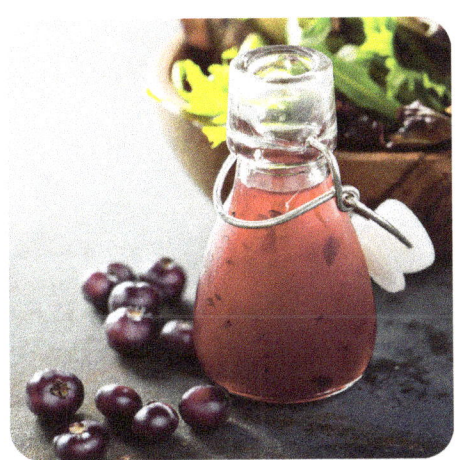

Cranberries' natural compounds (like proanthocyanidins) are know to support urinary tract health.

INGREDIENTS

½ cup	fresh cranberries
3 tbsp	extra virgin olive oil
3 tbsp	fresh orange juice
1.5 tbsp	fresh lemon juice
2 tbsp	organic red wine vinegar
4 med	fresh mint leaves
2 tbsp	raw coconut or agave nectar
¼ tsp	sea salt

SALAD INGREDIENTS:

12 ounces	arugula
1/2 cup	raw walnuts, chopped

Optional: 1 medium shallot or 1 small red onion, thinly sliced

DIRECTIONS

1. Add all ingredients, except mint to a food processor. Blend until smooth.
2. Add mint leaves and pulse for a few seconds.
3. Just before serving, drizzle vinaigrette over spinach, walnuts and shallots, until well distributed and spinach is well coated.
4. Serve immediately or refrigerate. Makes about ¾ to 1 cup of vinaigrette.

SERVINGS	TIME	LEVEL	KCAL	FIBER	CARB	FAT	PROTEIN
4-6	20 mins	easy	125	1g	8g	10g	0

Cranberry Maple Dressing
with Spinach Grape Salad

Tart cranberries and maple syrup blend with citrus and red wine vinegar for a sweet-sharp balance.

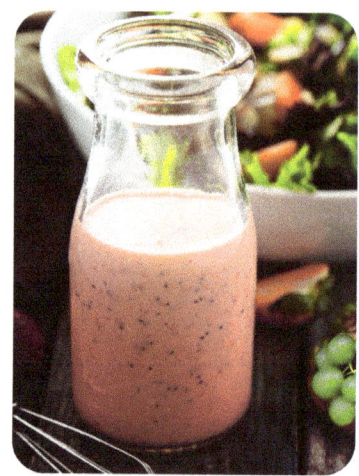

The natural pectin in cranberries gives this dressing a beautifully thick texture.

INGREDIENTS

½ cup	fresh cranberries
3 tbsp	extra virgin olive oil
3 tbsp	fresh orange juice
1 tbsp	fresh lemon juice
2 tbsp	organic red wine vinegar
2 tbsp	grade B, dark maple syrup
¼ tsp	sea salt

SALAD INGREDIENTS:

12 oz	fresh spinach
1 cup	red grapes, sliced in half
½ cup	raw pecans
1 med	shallot or 1 small red onion, thinly sliced

DIRECTIONS

1. Add all dressing ingredients to a food processor or blender and blend until smooth.
2. Just before serving, drizzle vinaigrette over spinach, grapes and shallots, until well distributed and spinach is well coated.
3. Serve immediately or refrigerate. Makes about 1 cup of vinaigrette.

SERVINGS	TIME	LEVEL	KCAL	FIBER	CARB	FAT	PROTEIN
4-8	20 mins	easy	162	1g	18g	10g	1g

Sweet Chili Sauce

Whip up this bold, tangy chili sauce in minutes, perfect for the collard green wraps, stir-fries, or as a marinade for tofu.

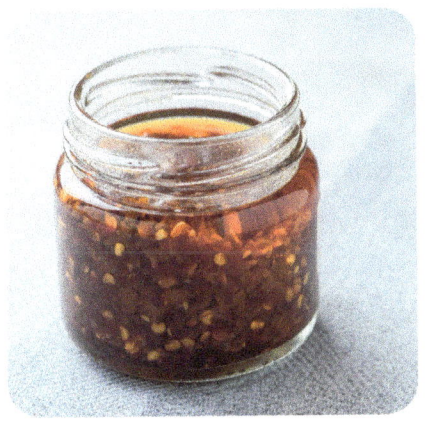

The vinegar and lime juice in this sauce act as natural preservatives, so it stays fresh for up to 3 weeks in the fridge.

INGREDIENTS

1/4 cup	brown rice vinegar
2 tbsp	water
2 tbsp	maple syrup
1 tbsp	tamari
1 inch	knob of ginger, minced
1 tsp	red pepper flakes, or to taste
1	lime, juiced
½ tsp	cayenne pepper or sriracha (adjust to heat preference)

DIRECTIONS

1. Add all sauce ingredients to a bowl and whisk until well mixed. If using a blender, add all ingredients except the chili flakes. Blend and then mix in chili flakes.
2. Store refrigerated for 2-3 weeks in an airtight container.

SERVINGS	TIME	LEVEL	KCAL	FIBER	CARB	FAT	PROTEIN
3	15 mins	easy	748	14g	54g	50g	30g

Peaceful Ranch Dressing

All the herby, tangy creaminess of the original, but just plants, no hormones, no cruelty, and no guilt.

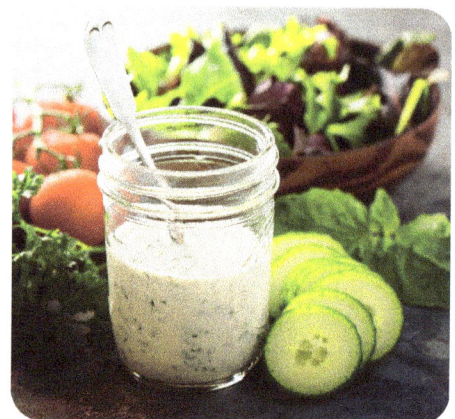

This ranch could convert a dairy diehard. But unlike traditional versions, it's rich in antioxidants like kaempferol (from parsley and dill), linked to reduced inflammation.

INGREDIENTS

1 cup	vegan mayo
¼ cup	coconut milk
1 tbsp	apple cider vinegar
1/2 tsp	lemon juice
2 tsp	flat-leaf parsley, finely chopped
1 tbsp	green onion, finely chopped
1 tsp	fresh dill, finely chopped
½ tsp	onion powder
½ tsp	garlic powder
¼ tsp	sea salt
¼ tsp	cracked pepper

DIRECTIONS

1. Whisk all ingredients together until smooth. Add more mayo to increase thickness or more coconut milk to make it thinner.
2. Adjust seasonings to taste.

SERVINGS	TIME	LEVEL	KCAL	FIBER	CARB	FAT	PROTEIN
6-8	20 mins	easy	513	0	3g	55g	1g

Coconut Sour Cream

Creamy, tangy, and dairy-free—this versatile topping upgrades tacos, soups, and baked potatoes with probiotic goodness.

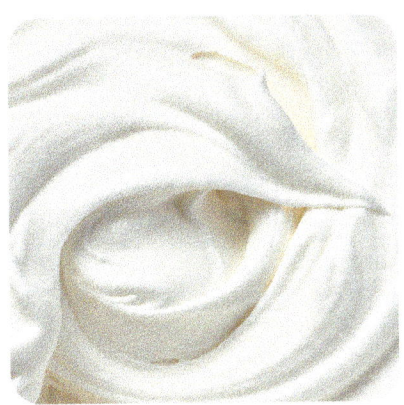

INGREDIENTS

6 ounces	organic coconut cream
1 tbsp	apple cider vinegar
1 tbsp	fresh lemon juice or lime juice
1/4 tsp	sea salt

Apple cider vinegar is made through fermentation, giving it natural probiotics and enzymes that support digestion and balance blood sugar.

DIRECTIONS

1. You can buy canned coconut cream, or you can place 1 can of regular (not light) coconut milk in the refrigerator for 4 or more hours. Open can and skim off solid portion (cream) of coconut milk. Save remaining liquid for use in a smoothie or some other recipe.
2. Whisk the coconut cream and remaining ingredients until smooth. Add a few tablespoons of the remaining coconut milk to loosen, if needed.
3. Serve immediately or store covered in the refrigerator for up to 5 days.

SERVINGS	TIME	LEVEL	KCAL	FIBER	CARB	FAT	PROTEIN
4-6	10 mins	easy	153	0	23g	7g	1g

Nacho Cheeze Sauce

Roasted red peppers and smoked paprika (non-negotiable!) blend with cashews into a velvety cheeze sauce; drench nachos, baked potatoes, or chili dogs, or swap it anywhere queso's needed.

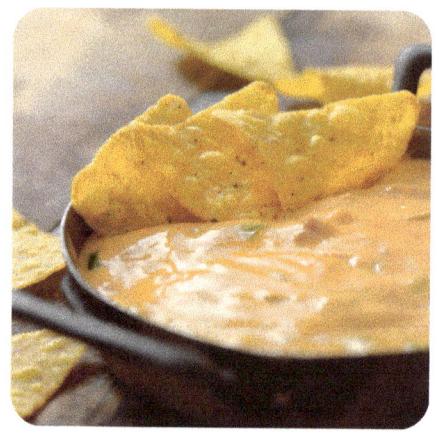

Smoked paprika's capsaicin may boost metabolism, while nutritional yeast adds gut-friendly B vitamins you can't get from dairy cheese.

INGREDIENTS

1 ½ cup	cashews, soaked for 2 hours or overnight, drained
1 large	red bell pepper (seeded)
3 tbsp	lemon juice
5 tbsp	nutritional yeast
1 tsp	sea salt (or to taste)
2 tbsp	**smoked** paprika
1/2 tsp	cayenne pepper or to taste
1/2 cup	water

DIRECTIONS

1. Add all ingredients, and 1/d of the water to the blender, beginning with the bell pepper for ease of blending.
2. Add water as needed to get mixture going.

SERVINGS	TIME	LEVEL	KCAL	FIBER	CARB	FAT	PROTEIN
5-8	20 mins	easy	**433**	7g	29g	31g	18g

Vegan Cotija Cheese

This "cheese" can be used as a delicious topping for salads, baked sweet potato, or other veggies.

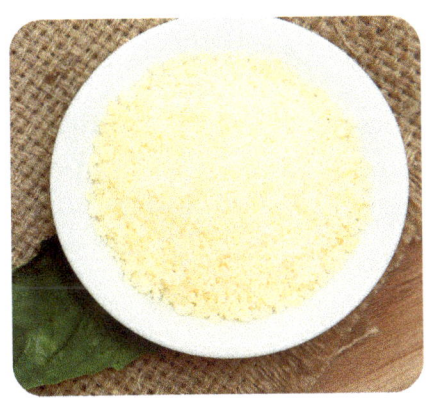

INGREDIENTS

1 cup	raw almonds
1/2	lemon, juiced (or 2 tbsp)
1	lime, juiced
1 tbsp	nutritional yeast
1 tsp	sea salt
1 tsp	garlic powder

Almonds are a great source of magnesium, which helps regulate blood sugar levels, supports muscle and nerve function, and promotes heart health.

DIRECTIONS

1. Pulse almonds in a food processor until ground into a powder.
2. Add all other ingredients and pulse or mix with smooth.
3. Use immediately or refrigerate for later use. Keeps well for 5-7 days.

Note: Make a double batch and freeze half for 1 month—this vegan cotija softens when thawed but still tastes sharp and salty, just like the fresh version.

SERVINGS	TIME	LEVEL	KCAL	FIBER	CARB	FAT	PROTEIN
8-16	10 mins	easy	115	3g	6g	9g	5g

Quick Vegan Parmesan

Cashews + nooch (nutritional yeast) = magic dust. Sprinkle this vegan parm on everything: salads, popcorn, roasted veggies, soup, avocado toast, even pizza.

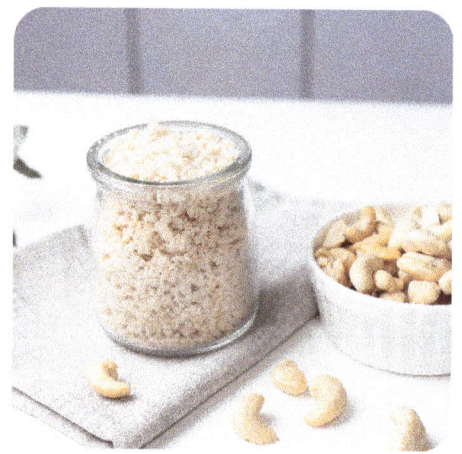

Nutritional yeast isn't just cheesy, it's a complete protein with B12, while hemp seeds add omega-3s.

INGREDIENTS

½ cup	raw cashews or raw pine nuts
½ cup	hemp seeds
¼ cup	sesame seeds
¼ cup	nutritional yeast
1 ½ tsp	garlic powder
1 tsp	sea salt or to taste

For a nut free version, sub raw sunflower seeds in place of cashews or pine nuts.

DIRECTIONS

1. Add all ingredients to a food processor. Pulse until you have fine powder.
2. Use immediately or store in the refrigerator for up to 2 weeks.

SERVINGS	TIME	LEVEL	KCAL	FIBER	CARB	FAT	PROTEIN
8-16	10 mins	easy	157	2g	8g	12g	7g

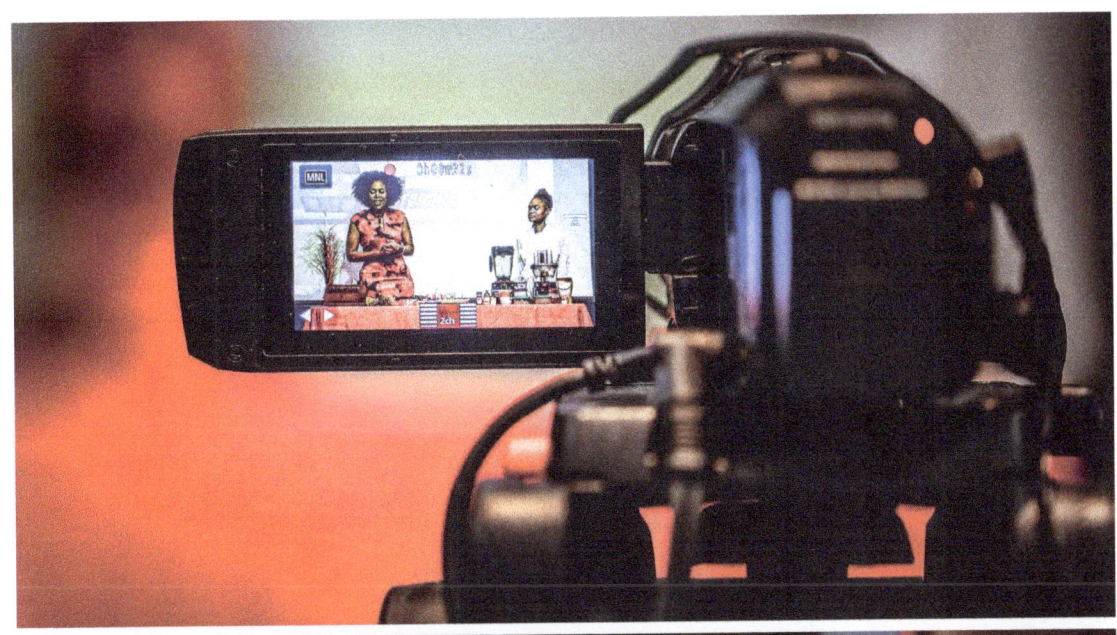

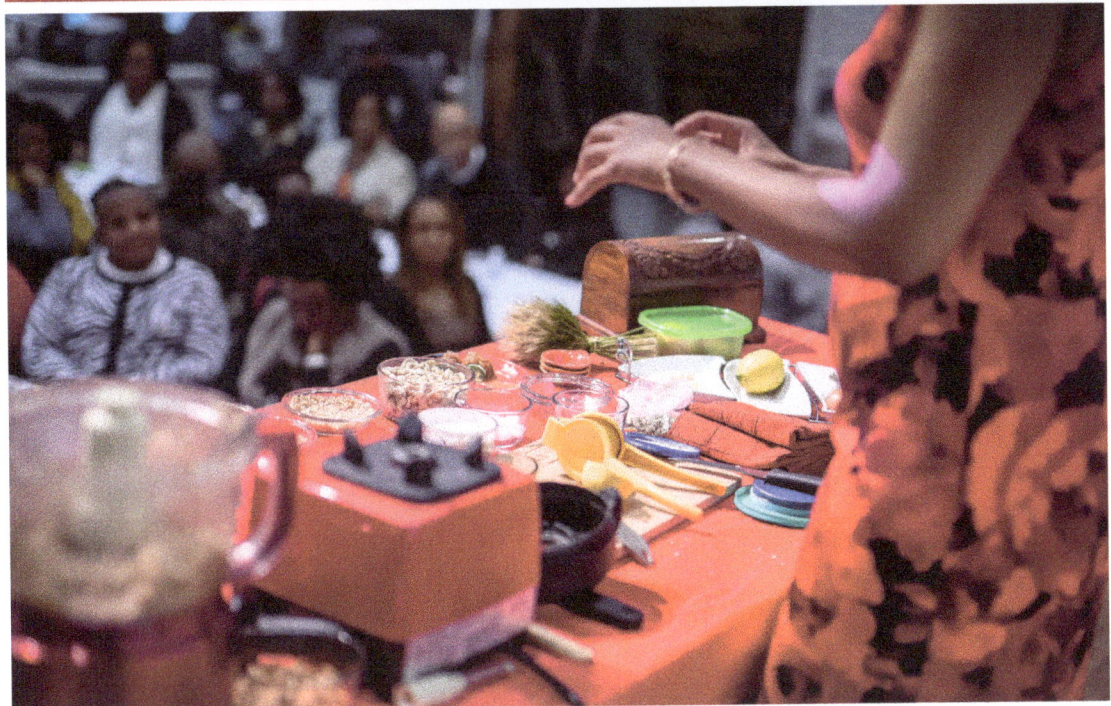

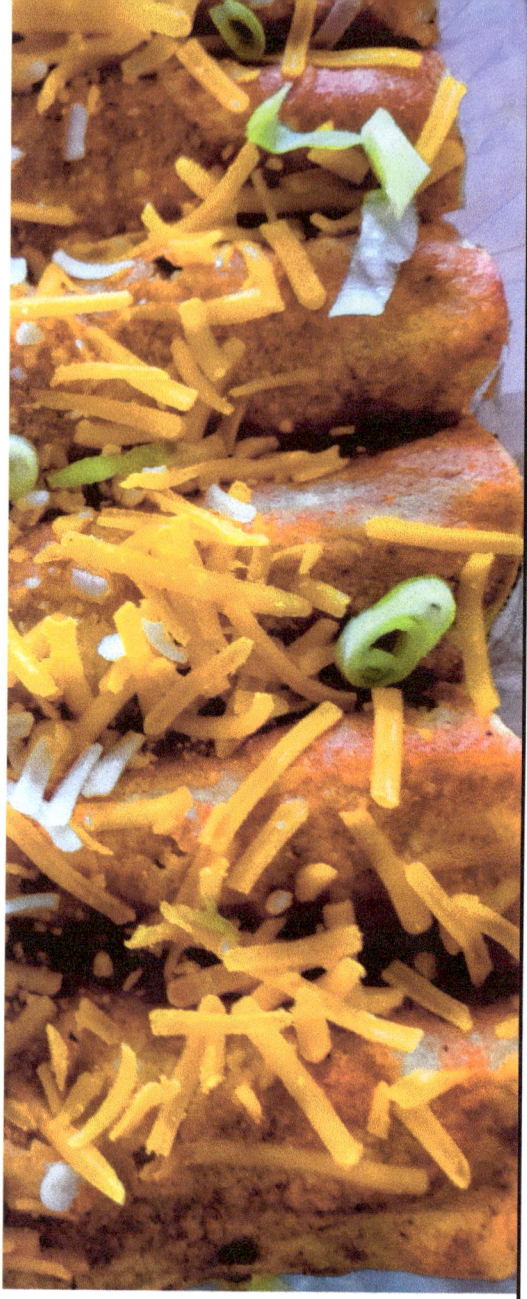

Splurge Smarter!

- 8 -
THE SPLURGE!

The Splurge!

Welcome to *The Splurge*, for the occasional indulgence. When I first went vegan, I thought all the decadent food that I loved was gone for good, like potato salad or a yummy grilled cheese sandwich. Then I discovered substitutes like cashew cheese, and my world changed! These recipes, like eggless savory quiche, velvety spinach fettuccini, and tempeh grilled cheese, prove that comfort food can be even more satisfying when it's made with whole ingredients. No deprivation, just satisfaction.

Like most people, I really loved cow's cheese, so this chapter is full of "cheezy" vegan dishes like the spinach basil manicotti, and the mac and cheese. These aren't just substitutes, they're revelations. Splurging shouldn't mean sacrificing taste or health.

(If you can't consume cashews, not to worry, firm tofu can often be used as a great replacement to achieve similar results.)

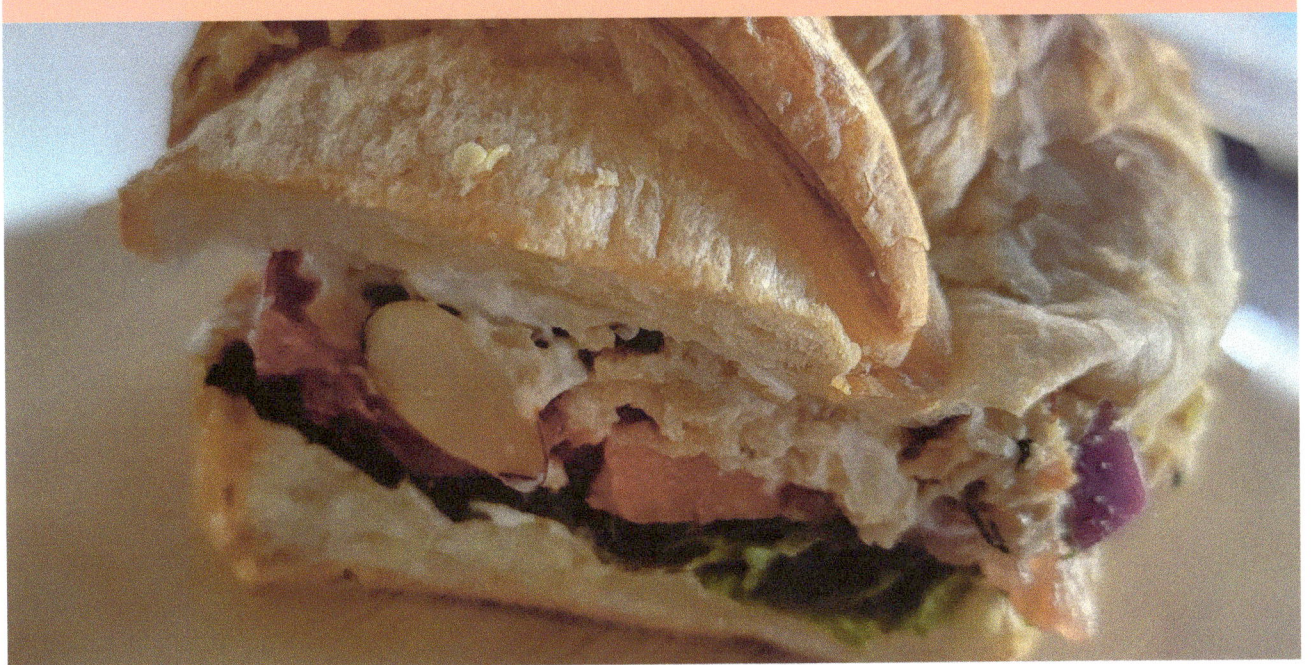

"Chicken" Salad on a Vegan Croissant

Cashew Crème Spinach Fettuccini

Creamy Alfredo sauce was my greatest vegan sacrifice... until I discovered blended cashews. Now, this luxuriously smooth pasta, tossed with garlicky spinach & mushrooms shows there's nothing to miss.

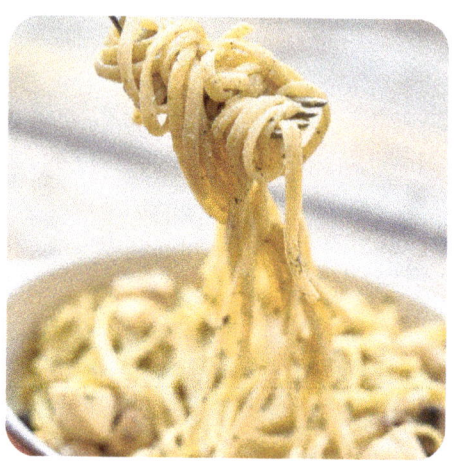

Cashews transform into velvety sauces because their healthy fats emulsify perfectly, while miso adds gut-friendly probiotics and a savory depth of flavor.

PASTA:
12 oz Spinach fettuccini pasta or other whole grain pasta

INGREDIENTS

1 cup	raw cashews
1 cup	hot water (best to use starchy pasta-cooking water)
1 tsp	fresh lemon juice
3	garlic cloves
1 tbsp	extra-virgin olive oil (optional)
2 tbsp	nutritional yeast
1 tsp	sea salt or to taste
1 tsp	white miso paste or tamari
1 tsp	paprika
½ tsp	cracked pepper or to taste
½ tsp	cayenne

VEGETABLES:

1	red or yellow bell pepper, chopped into 2-inch pieces
5 oz	baby spinach
1½ cup	baby bella mushrooms, sliced
2-3	shallots, thinly sliced

Continued on the next page.

SERVINGS	TIME	LEVEL	KCAL	FIBER	CARB	FAT	PROTEIN
4-5	45 mins	Intermediate	374	6g	31g	24g	14g

DIRECTIONS

1. Prepare pasta as directed on box. Cook pasta until it is al dente; it will continue cooking even after it is removed from the water. The longer you cook pasta the higher the glycemic index.
2. Place raw cashews in a food processor and pulse until nuts are very fine. Carefully add in the hot water; process until smooth.
3. Add the lemon juice, garlic, olive oil and nutritional yeast; process again until smooth.
4. Add sea salt and cracked pepper and adjust flavor with optional seasonings.
5. The blending process thickens the sauce; using starchy water helps this process. It may take few minutes to thicken. If it isn't thickening enough for you, heat it in a saucepan over a low temperature for a few minutes, and it will thicken.
6. In a large pan, sauté shallots, mushrooms and bell pepper in water until slightly softened. Mix in spinach and add cooked pasta.
7. Pour crème sauce over pasta and vegetables and mix until all ingredients are coated. Serve.

Feel free to add in your favorite vegetables.

This sauce is very versatile and can be used in a number of ways. It's a great topping for broccoli and a baked potato. It's also a great sauce for a vegetable stir fry.

Butternut Squash Lasagna

I love this twist on traditional lasagna. Butternut Squash Lasagna brings a creamy, hearty flavor with a fresh, veggie filling!

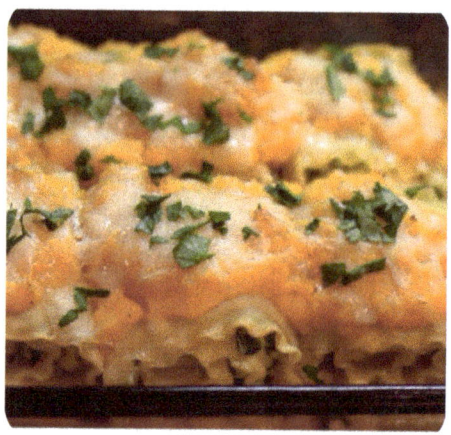

Butternut squash gets its vibrant orange color from beta-carotene, a carotenoid that the body converts into vitamin A to support immune function and eye health.

INGREDIENTS

12 oz box	gluten free lasagna noodles
3 cups	butternut squash, diced
5 cups	button mushrooms, sliced
15 oz	baby spinach
1 large	carrot, grated
2 cups	vegan mozzarella "cheese" shreds
2 tbsp	oregano, dried
2 tbsp	basil, dried

BUTTERNUT SAUCE INGREDIENTS:

3 cups	butternut squash, fresh or frozen, diced
13.5 oz	coconut milk, canned
1	red onion, rough chopped
4	cloves garlic
1 cup	basil
2 tsp	oregano
1 tsp	sage
1 tsp	sea salt
1 tsp	paprika
½ tsp	smoked paprika
½ tsp	cayenne
½ tsp	cracked pepper

Continued on the next page.

SERVINGS	TIME	LEVEL	KCAL	FIBER	CARB	FAT	PROTEIN
6	75 mins	intermediate	257	7g	29g	9g	18g

DIRECTIONS

1. Add all sauce ingredients except coconut milk to a sauce pan and sauté for 5-6 minutes. Add coconut milk and let simmer for 4 minutes.

2. With an immersion hand blender, carefully puree sauce (or carefully pour sauce into a blender and puree).

3. Evenly spread 1/3 butternut squash sauce on bottom of lasagna baking dish. Layer lasagna noodles on top of sauce.

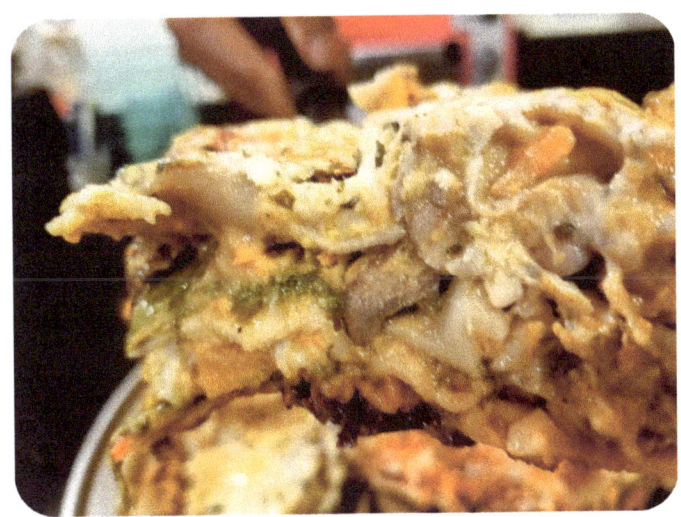

4. Add a layer of butternut squash over noodles; then add a layer of spinach, then add a layer of mushrooms.

5. Pour or ladle 1/3 of the butternut squash sauce over the mushrooms.

6. Add a layer of noodles, then shredded carrots, then spinach, then mushrooms, then a layer of vegan cheddar cheese shreds, then 1/3 of sauce.

7. Add a layer of noodles, any remaining veggies, and then a layer of sauce, then the remaining vegan cheddar cheese shreds.

8. Bake at 350°F for 45 minutes.

Veggie Lasagna with Cashew Ricotta

What I love most about lasagna is its flexibility. Choose your favorite veggies and start layering. Once I discovered the short cut of not boiling the lasagna noodles in advance, I started making lasagna a lot more often. Not only does skipping that step save time, it also increases the flavor by allowing the noodles to absorb the tomato sauce, rather than water. This dish is always a hit!

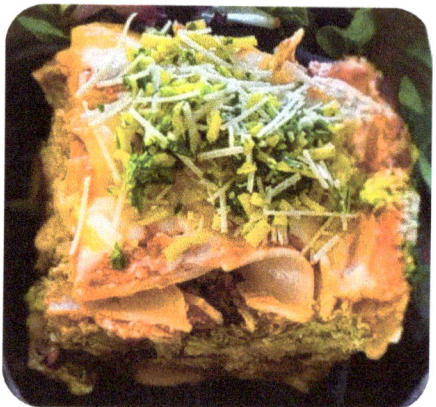

Firm tofu can be used in place of cashews for the ricotta--they both taste delicious!

INGREDIENTS

12 oz box	gluten free lasagna noodles
10 oz	baby spinach
3 cups	button mushrooms, sliced
3 cups	carrots, shredded
1 large	or 2 medium red onion(s), thinly sliced
2	red or orange bell peppers, sliced
1 cup	sundried tomatoes, chopped (rehydrate if dried)
16 oz	jar tomato sauce (Italian, basil, or mushroom works well)
8 oz	vegan mozzarella shreds
8 oz	vegan pepper jack shreds
1.5 cups	cashew basil ricotta (see page 117)
1 tbsp	dried parsley or 1/4 cup fresh parsley
1 tbsp	oregano or Italian seasoning
4 tbsp	nutritional yeast

Continued on the next page.

SERVINGS	TIME	LEVEL	KCAL	FIBER	CARB	FAT	PROTEIN
6-8	90 mins	intermediate	549	8g	64g	26g	22g

DIRECTIONS

Lasagna Assembly:
1. Base:
   - •Spread tomato sauce evenly across the bottom of a lasagna pan (9X13 inches).
2. First Layer Stack:
   - Onions: Cover entire dish with sliced red onions.
   - Noodles: Add uncooked lasagna noodles in a single layer.
   - Carrots: Scatter half the carrots over noodles.
   - Mushrooms: Add half the mushrooms.
   - Bell Peppers: Layer evenly.
   - Vegan Ricotta layer: Spread gently (use all contents on this layer)
   - Spinach: Distribute in an even layer. (use all contents on this layer)
   - Tomato sauce: Drizzle over spinach.
   - Nutritional yeast: Sprinkle 2 tbsp evenly.
   - Vegan cheese shreds: Mix vegan mozzarella and pepper jack shreds; layer on top.
   - Parsley: Sprinkle over cheese.
3. Repeat Layers:
   - Top with another layer of noodles, tomato sauce, then repeat with remaining onions, carrots, mushrooms, bell peppers, nutritional yeast & cheese shreds, parsley.
4. Final Toppings:
   - Add sundried tomatoes and remaining seasonings (oregano/Italian seasoning).
5. Baking:
   - Covered: Bake at 350°F for 35–40 minutes.
   - Uncovered: Bake 10–15 more minutes until bubbly.
   - Rest: Let cool for 15 minutes to firm up before serving.

Spinach Basil Manicotti

This rich classic was my ultimate comfort food hurdle as a vegan, until I cracked the vegan ricotta code. Now, these shells, stuffed with herbed spinach and mushrooms, then baked under a gooey vegan cheese blanket taste like victory.

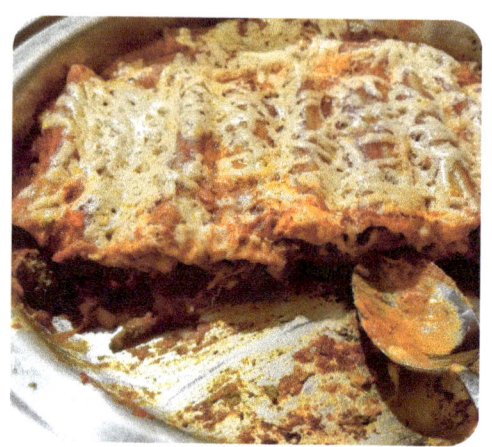

Cashew ricotta packs more protein and healthy fats than dairy ricotta, while basil's essential oils (like linalool) may help ease digestion.

INGREDIENTS

8 oz box	gluten-free Manicotti pasta noodles
16 oz	baby spinach
2 cups	button mushrooms
1 tbsp	oregano or Italian seasoning
24 oz	jar organic tomato sauce (Italian, basil, or mushroom work well)
8 oz	vegan cheddar "cheese" shreds

CASHEW BASIL RICOTTA INGREDIENTS

2 cups	raw cashews, soaked for 2-24 hours, drained (can sub 14oz of firm tofu)
¾ cup	fresh basil, packed, large stems removed
½ cup	water
1	lemon, juiced
3	garlic cloves
1 tsp	onion powder
½ tsp	sea salt
2 tbsp	nutritional yeast

Continued on the next page.

SERVINGS	TIME	LEVEL	KCAL	FIBER	CARB	FAT	PROTEIN
4-6	60 mins	intermediate	505	8g	44g	31g	23g

CASHEW BASIL RICOTTA DIRECTIONS:

1. Add cashews (or tofu), garlic, lemon juice, water, basil, nutritional yeast and onion powder to a food processor.
2. Pulse food processor until consistency looks like ricotta or cottage cheese, scraping down the sides as necessary. If the mixture is too dry, add a bit more water.
3. Season with sea salt & pepper to taste.
4. Set aside in a bowl.

MANICOTTI DIRECTIONS:

1. Place mushrooms and spinach in the food processor and pulse until mushroom are in small pieces.
2. Add mushrooms and spinach to the cashew ricotta and mix well.
3. In a casserole dish, spread ⅓ of the tomato sauce evenly across the bottom of the dish.
4. Stuff each hard shell (do not cook shells in advance) with the ricotta/mushroom stuffing using a small spoon, and gently place in the dish.
5. Top with the remaining tomato sauce so that all noodles are covered.
6. Top the cheese with the vegan cheddar cheese shreds, and Italian seasoning or oregano.
7. Bake, covered at 350°F for 35 minutes. Uncover and bake another 10-15 minutes. Let cool/rest for at least 10 minutes before serving (this gives it time to firm).

Baked Mac & Cheese

There are a million vegan mac & cheese recipes out there—this one is my easy, no-fuss favorite.

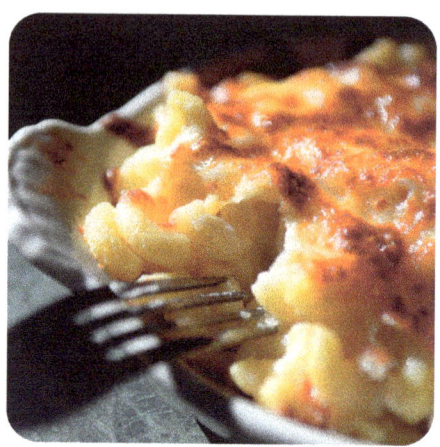

Button mushrooms bring umami depth and a meaty bite to this mac and cheese.

INGREDIENTS

16 oz	gluten-free elbow macaroni
8 oz	button mushrooms, roughly chopped
1½ cups	vegan cheddar cheese shreds

CHEESE SAUCE

1.5 cup	raw cashews, soaked 2 to 24 hours
3 tbsp	lemon juice
½ cup	nutritional yeast
2	garlic cloves
1 tsp	sea salt
1.5 tbsp	smoked paprika
1 tsp	cayenne pepper
½ cup	unsweetened light coconut milk

DIRECTIONS

1. Cook macaroni per instructions on box (cook al dente).
2. Add cheese sauce ingredients into a blender and blend until smooth.
3. Pour cheese sauce over pasta and mix until well incorporated.
4. Mix in 1 cup vegan cheddar cheese shreds and chopped mushrooms until well incorporated.
5. Oil or spray a baking dish with olive or coconut oil. Add contents to baking dish.
6. Top with ½ cup of vegan cheddar cheese shreds.
7. Bake for 30 minutes at 375°F until cheese has melted.

SERVINGS	TIME	LEVEL	KCAL	FIBER	CARB	FAT	PROTEIN
8 -10	50 mins	easy	355	7g	29g	21g	18g

Green Chile Enchiladas

Green please! That's my answer to the New Mexico state question: "Red or green?" While living in Albuquerque, NM, I developed an infinity for green chiles; it's added to everything, from chocolate to scones! The more I had it, the more I loved it. I certainly had green chile withdrawals when I moved away. This is my culinary ode to New Mexico, the beloved chile and all the wonderful friends I've met there.

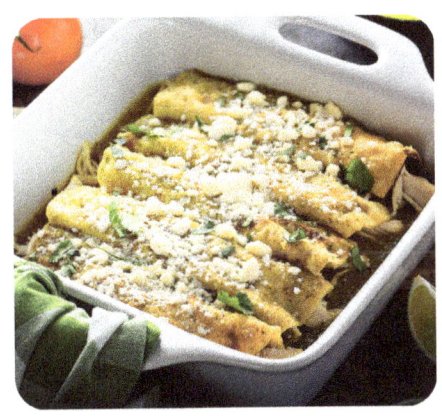

New Mexico's Hatch green chiles have their own trademark, and their earthy-sweet flavor elevates any dish.

INGREDIENTS

12-16	medium tortillas (corn or whole grain)
½ pound	portobello mushrooms, cleaned & sliced
5 cups	baby spinach, packed
2 cups	pinto beans, cooked
2 cups	vegan pepper jack cheese shreds, divided in half (or use Nacho Cheeze, page 105)
1	onion, diced
½ cup	cilantro, chopped
8 oz	green chiles, chopped

ENCHILADA SAUCE:

6 med	tomatillos
1 med	tomato, vine ripened or Roma
1 large	jalapeno pepper, seeds removed
8 oz	green chiles
14 oz	coconut milk
½ cup	water
1 med	shallot or red onion
2 cloves	garlic
1 tsp	sea salt

Continued on the next page.

SERVINGS	TIME	LEVEL	KCAL	FIBER	CARB	FAT	PROTEIN
4-6	55 mins	intermediate	345	5g	20g	26g	13g

Green Chile Enchiladas - *continued*

DIRECTIONS

1. Pre-heat oven to 375°F.
2. In a skillet or large sauce pan, sauté the mushrooms, spinach, beans, onion, and green chilies for about 5-7 minutes.
3. Add in the cilantro and half the cheese and sauté until the cheese melts, 2-3 minutes. Turn off heat.
4. Blend enchilada sauce ingredients in a blender. Blend until smooth.
5. Pour enough enchilada sauce in a baking dish to cover the bottom of the dish (9x13 inches).
6. Spoon about 1/12 of the mixture onto a tortilla and roll it up and place it, seam side down into the baking dish. Roll the other tortillas and place side by side in baking dish.
7. Pour the remaining enchilada sauce over the tortillas and sprinkle with the remaining cheese.
8. Bake at 375°F for 30 minutes, until tortillas are heated through.
9. Serve with Coconut Sour Cream (see page 104) and guacamole or avocado slices. You can also top with vegan Cotija Cheese (see page 106).

Super Veg Pizza with Cashew Cheese

This is the pizza that made me stop missing dairy-based pizza. This pizza is so rich and satisfying; you will devour it!

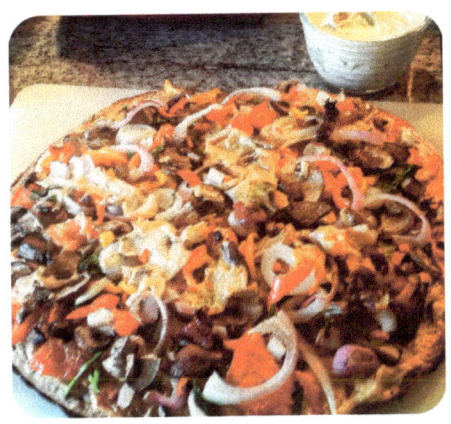

Sundried tomatoes have 10x the lycopene (a potent antioxidant) of fresh tomatoes.

INGREDIENTS

1	whole wheat or gluten pizza crust
1 cup	cashew cheese (recipe on page 82)
2 medium	vine ripened or Roma tomatoes
1/4 cup	sundried tomatoes, chopped
1 cup	spinach, chopped
1 cup	button mushrooms, sliced
1 large	shallot, sliced
5 mini	bell peppers or ½ red or yellow bell pepper
1 tbsp	olive oil
2 tbsp	fresh or dried oregano
2 tbsp	fresh or dried basil
½ tsp	sea salt
dash	cracked pepper, to taste

DIRECTIONS

1. Bake pizza crust at 425°F for 5-7 minutes, remove, let cool for 3-4 minutes.
2. Spoon a thick layer or cashew cheese onto crust, spread evenly
3. Sprinkle half oregano and basil over cheese .
4. Place thinly sliced tomatoes side by side until crust is completely covered. Drizzle or brush with olive oil and sprinkle with sea salt
5. Add chopped spinach, onions, mushrooms, peppers, shallots and sundried tomatoes evenly over pizza.
6. Top with remaining oregano, basil and sea salt.
7. Spoon a few small dollops of cashew cheese on top and spread gently over pizza. Drizzle with remaining olive oil. Top with cracked pepper.
8. Bake at 400°F for 10-12 minutes until slightly browned. Serve immediately.

SERVINGS	TIME	LEVEL	KCAL	FIBER	CARB	FAT	PROTEIN
4	45 mins	intermediate	221	8g	39g	6g	8g

Tempeh Grilled Cheese

The grilled cheese upgrade! Smoky tempeh, melty nacho cheese, and caramelized shallots smash between toasty sprouted grain bread for a sandwich that's crispy, gooey, and deeply satisfying.

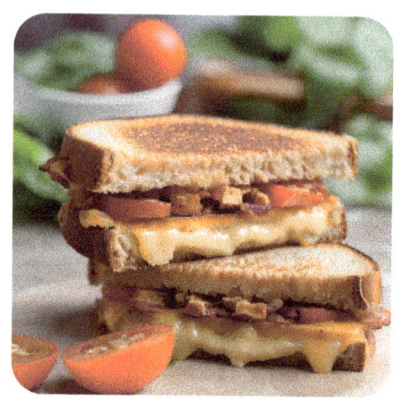

INGREDIENTS

1 cup	nacho cheeze (recipe on page 105)
1	shallot or 1/2 medium red onion
1 med	tomato
8 oz	maple flavored tempeh strips or tempeh bacon
6	slices sprouted grain bread
3 tbsp	coconut oil

Tempeh's fermentation process boosts protein digestibility, while sprouted grain bread offers more bioavailable nutrients than regular bread. This is comfort food that works for you.

DIRECTIONS

1. Sauté onions and tempeh for 3-5 minutes with 1 tablespoon coconut oil over medium heat.
2. Remove from pan and set aside.
3. Spread coconut oil on both sides of the bread and put 2 slices in the hot pan. Let heat and brown for few minutes, flipping to brown both sides.
4. Spread 1-2 tablespoons nacho cheeze to bread carefully, add onion and then tempeh slices, top with 2 tomato slices. Add 1 tablespoon to other side of bread and close sandwich. Press down gently until heated through. Flip and let heat the other side for 1 minute (optional).

Serving Suggestion: Serve with avocado on the side and a creamy coleslaw.

SERVINGS	TIME	LEVEL	KCAL	FIBER	CARB	FAT	PROTEIN
3	30 mins	easy	591	8g	47g	31g	32g

"Chicken" Salad Sliders

These sliders are my party secret, vegan 'chicken,' crunchy celery, sweet grapes, and a tangy dill-mayo dressing make this a winner. Trust me on the grape-and-almond combo!

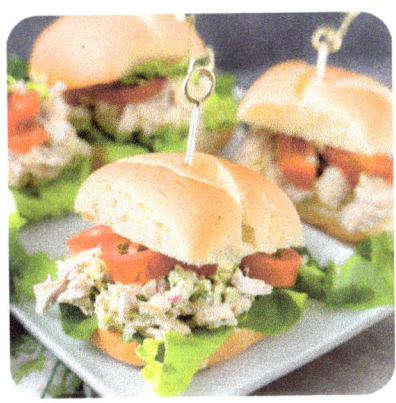

Don't skip the dill!, its a game changer for this recipe & may also aid digestion.

INGREDIENTS

12 oz	vegan chicken nugget/patties (soy)
2 ribs	celery, diced
2	green onions, chopped
½	red onion, sliced
½ cup	red grapes, sliced
3 tbsp	fresh dill, chopped
⅓ cup	sliced almonds
¼ cup	vegan mayo
1 tbsp	apple cider vinegar or lemon juice
1 tbsp	Dijon mustard
pinch	sea salt & pepper to taste
4	butter or green leaf lettuce leaves
6-8	slider buns or soft rolls

DIRECTIONS

1. Cook vegan chick'n tender in oven for 20 minutes on 375°F. For vegan chick'n packed in liquid, sauté in pan for 15 minutes until browned, over medium heat.
2. Add celery, onion and dill to food processor and pulse into small pieces. Place ingredients in large mixing bowl.
3. Add chick'n to food processor and pulse until it is in bite size pieces. Add chick'n to the bowl.
4. Add mayo, mustard and apple cider vinegar to the bowl. Mix well. Adjust seasoning to taste. Add a pinch of sea salt and pepper to taste.
5. Add mayo to slidier bun then lettuce, tomato & chick'n salad and top bun.

SERVINGS	TIME	LEVEL	KCAL	FIBER	CARB	FAT	PROTEIN
3	30 mins	easy	608	5g	38g	23g	45g

Baked Buffalo Cauliflower Wings

Cauliflower that bites back. These florets bring the heat—and the fiber, and the antioxidants… but mostly the heat. 🌶️

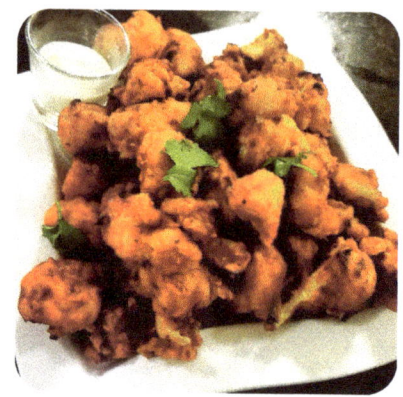

Capsaicin (the fire in your hot sauce) may boost circulation & metabolism.

INGREDIENTS

1 head	cauliflower (approx. 5 cups of florets)
1 cup	light coconut milk
1 cup	all-purpose gluten-free flour
3 tbsp	garlic powder
1 tsp	cumin
1 tsp	onion powder
2 tsp	of smoked paprika
½ tsp	sea salt
¼ tsp	cracked pepper
1 cup	buffalo wing sauce (i.e.,Primal Kitchen Buffalo Sauce)

DIRECTIONS

1. Preheat oven to 425°F. Line baking sheet with natural un-bleached parchment paper or spray with coconut oil spray. If using oil, be sure to coat the baking sheet well with oil or cauliflower will stick.
2. Wash and cut cauliflower head into bite size pieces.
3. Mix the coconut milk, flour and spices in a large mixing bowl (set the hot sauce aside for later). Mix until the batter is thick and can coat the cauliflower.
4. Dip the cauliflower in the batter. Shake off excess batter. Lay florets in single layer on baking sheet.
5. Bake for 30 minutes until golden brown. Flip florets over half way through the baking to get all sides crispy.
6. After cauliflower has baked for 30 minutes, remove from oven and put baked florets into a mixing bowl with the wing sauce and toss until evenly coated.
7. Return cauliflower to baking sheet and bake for an additional 20-25 minutes. Serve as-is, or with vegan ranch (recipe on page 103), or vegan blue cheese.

SERVINGS	TIME	LEVEL	KCAL	FIBER	CARB	FAT	PROTEIN
3-4	60 min	easy	372	6g	48g	18g	11g

Eggless/Crustless Savory Quiche

Chickpea flour's binding power (due to its high protein & starch) makes this quiche hold together without eggs, while cashews add creaminess.

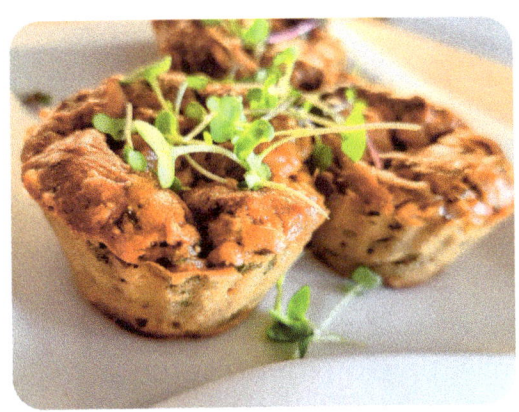

INGREDIENTS

2 cups	cashews (soaked for 2 hours or overnight)
¾ cup	chickpea flour
1 tbsp	baking powder
1 tsp	baking soda
1 tsp	cayenne
1/2 tsp	paprika
2 tbsp	nutritional yeast
3-4	sundried tomatoes, chopped
½ tsp	sea salt
2-3	garlic cloves
¼ cup	water

No time to soak? A quick 10-minute warm water soak softens cashews for easier blending.

VEGGIES:

3 cups	spinach, chopped
1	red onion, diced
1	red bell pepper, diced
1 cup	button or cremini mushrooms, diced

DIRECTIONS

1. Preheat oven to 325°F. Oil muffin pan with olive oil spray.
2. Drain and rinse soaked cashews. Add cashews and all base ingredients to a blender; blend until mixture is smooth. It will be very thick.
3. Lightly sauté all veggies, medium heat for 3 minutes. Remove from heat.
4. Pour sauce over veggies and mix until well incorporated.
5. With an ice cream scooper, evenly scoop mixture into a muffin pan.
6. Bake at 325 F for 50 minutes. Let cool. Makes about 12 muffin-sized quiches. Serving Suggestion: Serve with an arugula/red onion salad.

SERVINGS	TIME	LEVEL	KCAL	FIBER	CARB	FAT	PROTEIN
4-6	90 mins	advanced	600	8g	44g	41g	23g

Yellow Grits with Leeks & Mushrooms

Growing up in Alabama, grits were a delicious staple on the weekends. This version stays true to that soul-warming goodness, just lightly elevated with buttery leeks, savory mushrooms, and a sprinkle of vegan parm.

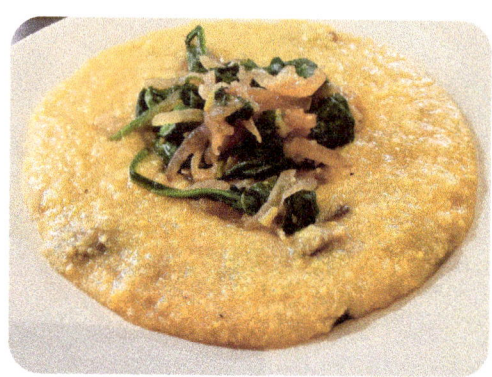

Stone-ground yellow grits retain more fiber and nutrients than instant versions.

INGREDIENTS

3 cups	water
1 cup	organic yellow grits
1 large	leek, sliced
1 cup	mushrooms, sliced
¼ cup	vegan parmesan (recipe on page 107)
3 tbsp	tamari, dvided
2 tsp	coconut oil (optional)
1 tsp	smoked paprika
½-¾ tsp	sea salt
¼ tsp	cayenne pepper
½	avocado, sliced

DIRECTIONS

1. In a medium sauce pan, bring water to boil.
2. Slowly stir in salt, tamari and grits to prevent lumps and mix well.
3. Bring to boil and then turn down to a simmer, stirring occasionally.
4. Simmer for 5 minutes and then remove from heat.
5. While grits are cooking, sauté leeks and mushrooms for 3-5 minutes, in 1-2 tbsp water or in coconut oil and ½ tsp paprika and 1 tbsp tamari.
6. Serve grits topped with a heaping tablespoon of vegan parmesan, and a large spoon full of leeks and mushrooms and a few slices of avocado.

SERVINGS	TIME	LEVEL	KCAL	FIBER	CARB	FAT	PROTEIN
2-4	20 mins	easy	151	4g	12g	22g	3g

Mushroom Tart with
Potato & Black-eyed Pea Crust

I debuted this tart at one of my annual Thanksgiving dinner/cooking class—and it stole the show I was looking for a gluten-free crust and this worked great.

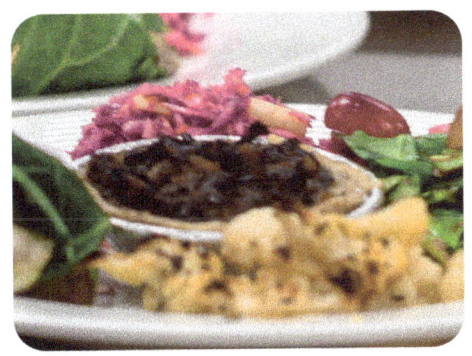

Black-eyed peas have more protein and fiber than traditional flour crusts, and their natural starch helps bind the potatoes without gluten.

CRUST INGREDIENTS:

1 ½ cups	cooked black-eyed peas
2 med	potatoes, boiled
3	garlic cloves, minced
1 tsp	sea salt
½ tsp	onion powder
¼ tsp	cayenne

FILLING INGREDIENTS

1 ½ cups	mushrooms, shitake or button
10 oz	spinach, coarsely chopped
¼ cup	coconut milk, canned (full fat)
2 large	onions, thinly sliced
1/2 cup	parsley, chopped
2 tbsp	water
2 tbsp	coconut amino or tamari
2 tbsp	arrowroot powder (to thicken)
½ tsp	sea salt
½ tsp	cracked pepper

Continued on the next page.

SERVINGS	TIME	LEVEL	KCAL	FIBER	CARB	FAT	PROTEIN
4-6	60 mins	intermediate	268	9g	47g	5g	14g

DIRECTIONS

CRUST:

1. Add cooked potatoes, cooked black-eyed peas and other crust ingredients into a food processor
2. Pulse in a food processor until somewhat smooth and all ingredients are well mixed. Place in refrigerator until cool enough to touch with hands, about 20 minutes.
3. After mixture has cooled, press into a 8-inch round or square baking dish, or put 2-3 tablespoons and press into individual tart pans.

FILLING:

1. Preheat oven to 350°F. Place onions and 2 tbsp water into a large pan and sauté for about 5 minutes, until onions become soft.
2. Add mushrooms to pan and sauté for another 5 minutes until mushrooms begin to cook down.
3. Add sea salt and tamari and mix well. Add coconut milk and bring to low boil; turn down to a simmer.
4. Add spinach until it wilts. Mixture should be very thick.
5. Pour mixture onto crust and smooth evenly. Bake for 35 minutes. Serve warm.

Boiling & Peeling Potatoes:

Peel 2 medium potatoes. Cut into even chunks for faster cooking. Boil in salted water for 10-15 mins until fork-tender. Drain and let cool slightly before mashing.

Cooking Black-Eyed Peas for this recipe (if using canned: drain &rinse):

Stovetop: Rinse 1 cup dried black-eyed peas. Add peas and 2.5 cups of water (no salt) to a pot. Bring to boil, then simmer, partially covered for 30-45 mins until tender. Then drain and rinse.

Roasted Stuffed Tomatoes and Peppers

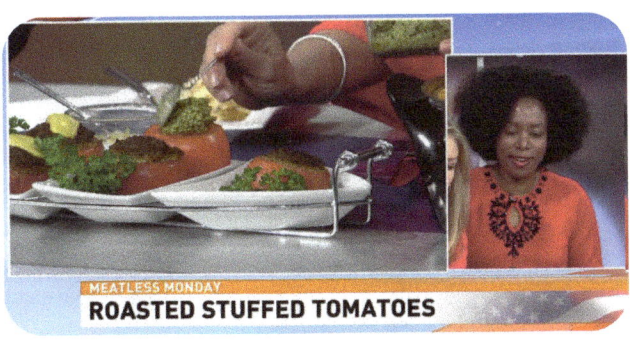

ROASTED STUFFED TOMATOES

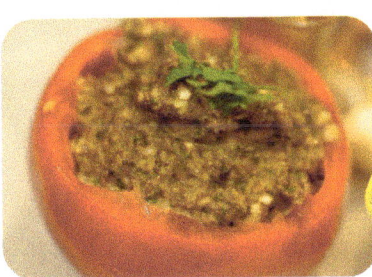

Serve these as a side or a light main with crusty bread.

INGREDIENTS

6 med   vine-ripened tomatoes
8 mini   bell peppers

FILLING INGREDIENTS

1.5 cups	mushrooms, button & shitake
1 cup	spinach, chopped
3/4 cup	cashews
3 tbsp	nutritional yeast
2 tbsp	olive oil
1 tbsp	tamari
1 small	red onion
2	garlic cloves
3/4 cup	parsley
½ tsp	sea salt
½ tsp	basil

DIRECTIONS

1. Cut a thin slice (about ½ inch) off the top of the tomatoes. Remove pulp and set aside in a bowl.
2. Slice the mini bell pepper in half, lengthwise and discard the core and seeds.
3. Put 3 tablespoons of the tomato pulp into a food processor along with all other filling ingredients.
4. Pulse the food processor until all ingredients are well mixed.
5. With a small spoon, stuff each of the tomatoes & mini peppers with the stuffing.
6. Refrigerate mini bell peppers until ready to serve.
7. Place the stuffed tomatoes in a baking dish and bake at 350°F for 30-minutes. Serve warm.

SERVINGS	TIME	LEVEL	KCAL	FIBER	CARB	FAT	PROTEIN
6	50 mins	intermediate	409	5g	27g	30g	15g

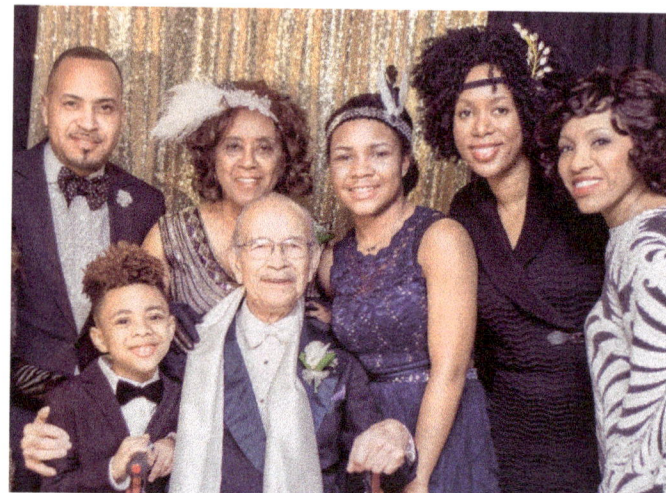

Family Time

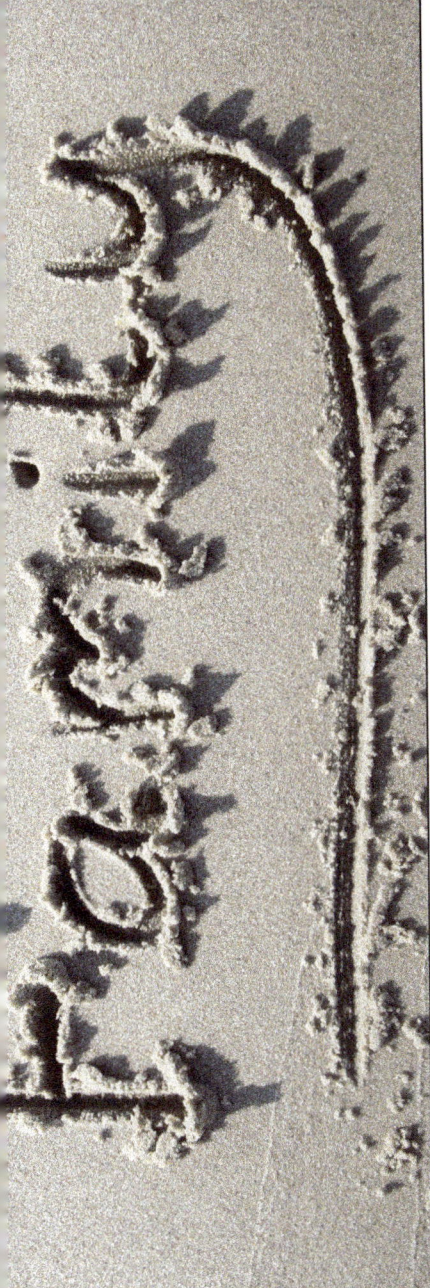

Love served on every plate.

- 9 -
FAMILY AFFAIR

Family Affair

Food has always been the heartbeat of our family, a way to pass down love, laughter, and the occasional friendly debate. This chapter is a tribute to those moments, with dishes that carry our stories. Mom's Vegan 'Beef' Wellington is a holiday showstopper she perfected after we went vegetarian, then vegan. The family went mostly vegan after my thyroid cancer recovery, which was why I went vegan. Dad's Peas & Rice was born from our years in the Bahamas. And my Aunt Ruby's (who I'm named after) Sweet Potato Pie? That's pure soul food alchemy.

What ties these recipes together isn't just the ingredients—it's the intention behind them. Marcus's Sweet Heat Nachos are a game-day essential. Michael's BBQ Meatballs are so perfected, even meat lovers request them. And Erika's Eggplant Parmesan is proof that good food can be made simply. Our recipes are our family heirlooms. Cook them, tweak them, and maybe even start a few new family traditions of your own.

In order: Sister, Mom, Niece, Me, Brother, Brother, Nephew & Niece

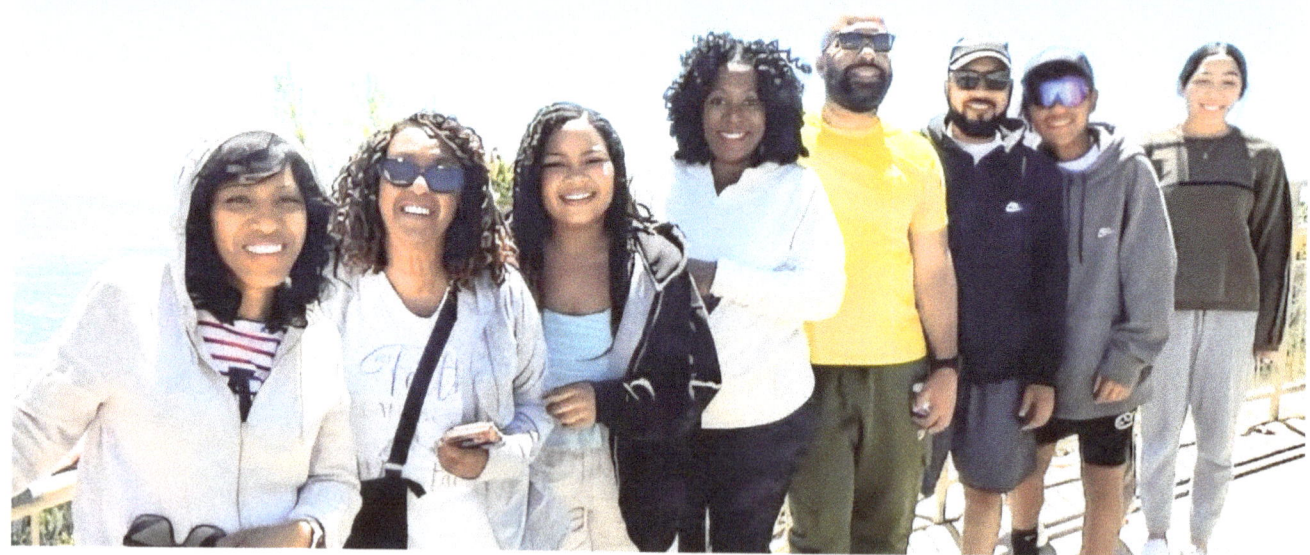

Mom's Vegan "Beef" Wellington

I learned to cook by watching my mother and then helping in the kitchen. When the family became vegetarian, she came up with lots of vegetarian and vegan versions of dishes. This is one of our family's favorites especially for Sabbath dinners or holidays. It is a delightful, heartwarming dish, always made with love, my mom's secret ingredient.

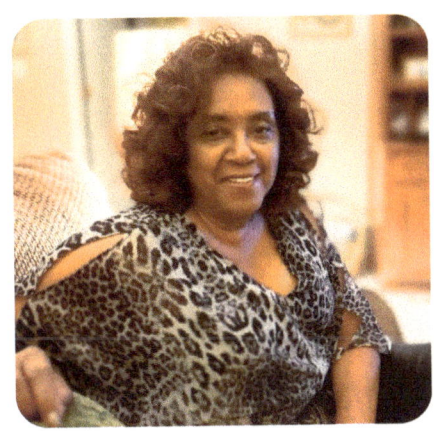

INGREDIENTS

10 oz	Beyond Meat "Beef" Crumbles, vegan
½ cup	Earth Balance Buttery Spread
8 oz	portabella mushrooms, chopped
1 med	green pepper, finely chopped
1 med	onion, finely chopped
½ tsp	garlic powder
½ tsp	Italian seasoning
¼ tsp	thyme

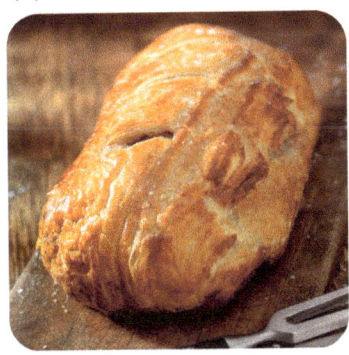

Textured Veg Protein (TVP) or more cooked lentils can be subbed for the "beef" crumbles.

DIRECTIONS

1. Make curst first and place in refrigerator for 30 minutes.
2. Preheat oven to 375ºF.
3. Add vegan butter to cooking pan, add chopped onion, green pepper, portabella mushrooms the vegan beef crumbles and seasonings. Sauté over medium heat until brown and vegetables are soft and caramelized.
4. Let cool. Spread the "meat" mixture on top of the prepared crust.
5. Once the meat mixture has been smoothed out over the crust you can begin to roll the crust and mixture in the same fashion as you would a cinnamon roll bun. Tuck in or trim the loose edges of crust.
6. Transfer to a baking sheet & bake for 45 minutes or until crust is a golden brown.
7. To serve, slice the Wellington into thick pieces and serve with the red wine sauce.

Continued on the next page.

SERVINGS	TIME	LEVEL	KCAL	FIBER	CARB	FAT	PROTEIN
6	20 mins	Advanced	269	2g	10g	14g	25g

Wellington Crust & Red Wine Sauce - *continued*

CRUST INGREDIENTS

2 cups	all-purpose unbleached flour sifted
½ cup	**cold** vegan butter, cut into small pieces
¼ tsp	sea salt
½ tsp	coconut sugar
2 tbsp	coconut oil
7-8 tbsp	ice water

RED WINE SAUCE INGREDIENTS

1 tbsp	olive oil
1 large	shallot, minced
1 ½ cups	dry red wine
1/2 cup	vegetable broth
4 tbsp	unsalted vegan butter, cold
pinch	sea salt & pepper, to taste

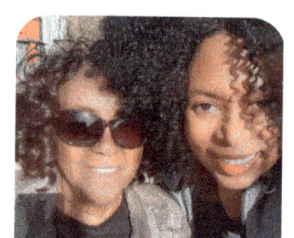

CRUST DIRECTIONS

1. Combine flour (can sub *all-purpose* gluten free flour), sugar, and salt in large bowl, mix well.
2. Add vegan butter (i.e., Earth Balance, Miyoko's Creamery) and oil to flour mixture and mix with fingers or pastry blender until you have pea-size pieces.
3. Sprinkle 5 to 6 tablespoons of ice water over the flour mixture and work the dough until it comes together in a ball. Only add the remaining tablespoons of water if necessary.
4. Make into a ball, wrap in plastic wrap and place in the refrigerator for 30 minutes.
5. Remove from refrigerator and place on floured surface and sprinkle flour on top of ball.
6. Use a rolling pin to roll out the crust to less the ¼ inch. The crust should be spread in an oblong shape for rolling (approximately 12 x 15 inches in size).

RED WINE SAUCE DIRECTIONS

1. Heat the oil in a medium sauté pan and add the shallot. Cook for about 5 mins over medium heat until soft and golden. Add the red wine, increase the heat to med/high and cook until the wine is reduced by about 2/3. Add the broth and continue to cook for another five minutes.
2. Strain the sauce using a fine mesh strainer and discard the solids. Return the sauce to the pan over medium heat.
3. Swirl in the butter one pat at a time until each piece is fully dissolved. Season with sea salt & pepper. Sauce should be slightly thickened and glossy.

Dad's Peas & Rice

My dad picked up most of his cooking skills from my mom. The story goes, he only knew how to make 2 or 3 dishes when they met!😂 He learned a lot over the years and whipped up some great meals. He came up with this dish with inspiration from the years that we lived in the Bahamas, where peas and rice is a staple. Though he's no longer here, this dish keeps his spirit at our table.

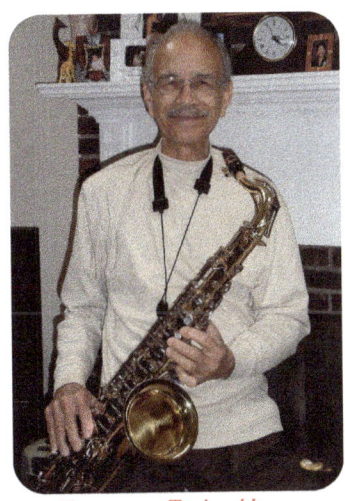

James F. Lathon

INGREDIENTS

1 cup	brown rice
1 cup	cooked black beans or kidney beans
2 cups	water (sub coconut milk for extra richness)
½ small	onion
2 tbsp	coconut oil
1 tbsp	*McKay's Vegan Chicken Style Instant Broth & Seasoning*
1 tsp	organic curry powder
¼ tsp	Cajun seasoning

Peas & rice form a complete protein, while coconut oil's fats help absorb curry's anti-inflammatory curcumin— island wisdom at work!

DIRECTIONS

1. Heat oil in small pan over medium heat.
2. Add finely chopped onion to pan and sauté until soft; don't let brown or burn.
3. Pour in 1 cup of water. Add 1 cup of rice and stir.
4. Mix in curry powder, Cajun seasoning and McKay's broth.
5. Stir and add 1 cup of water.
6. Reduce heat to low and cook for 30 minutes or until water is gone.

SERVINGS	TIME	LEVEL	KCAL	FIBER	CARB	FAT	PROTEIN
4	45 mins	easy	299	6g	48g	8g	8g

Erika's Easy Eggplant Parmesan

Erika likes to keep cooking simple, quick and yummy!

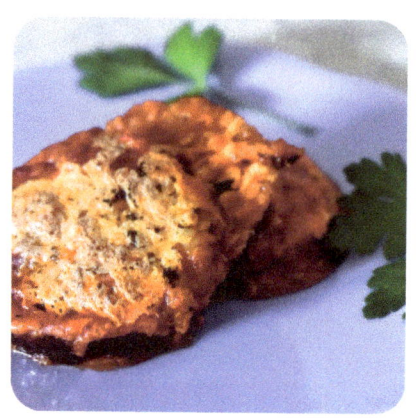

INGREDIENTS

1 large	eggplant or 2 medium eggplants, sliced
25 oz	marinara sauce (1 jar)
2 cups	vegan "mozzarella" cheese shreds
1 ½ cups	vegan bread crumbs
2 tbsp	olive oil, for brushing eggplant slices

Serving suggestion: Add spaghetti on the side, with the remaining marinara sauce--great with steamed broccoli or a salad.

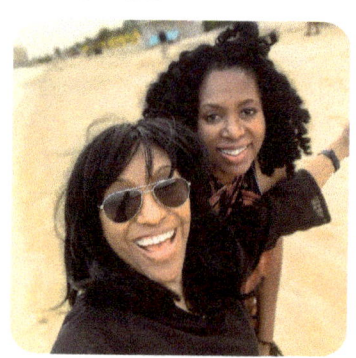

DIRECTIONS

1. Preheat oven to 375°F.
2. Slice eggplant into ½ inch round slices and brush with olive oil.
3. Bake for about 10 minutes and the flip eggplant and bake for another 15 minutes.
4. Put layer marinara sauce (about 1/3 cup) in bottom of a casserole dish (9X9 or larger) and spread evenly.
5. Add a single layer of the baked eggplant.
6. Add a layer of bread crumbs, about ½ cup.
7. Add a layer vegan shredded cheese.
8. Repeat layers until casserole is full, end cheese and then top with about ¼ cup of breadcrumbs.
9. Bake until casserole is heated &cheese is melted, about 35-40 minutes.

SERVINGS	TIME	LEVEL	KCAL	FIBER	CARB	FAT	PROTEIN
3-4	55 mins	easy	467	10g	55g	13g	10g

Erika's Spicy Sweet Potato Casserole

This is certainly a comfort dish! My sister, Erika is a healthy eater, mostly cooking light and yummy stir-fries, pastas with rich tomato sauces and always plenty of veggies. Occasionally she makes a decadent, but easy, dish such as this yummy casserole--a fam favorite!

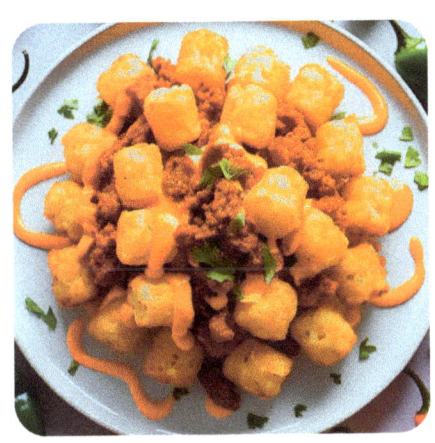

INGREDIENTS

32 oz sweet potato tots/puffs

12 oz vegan chorizo (such as Soyrizo Meatless Soy Chorizo or Sprouts Soy Chorizo)

1 cup vegan cheddar cheese shreds or use Nacho Cheeze Recipe on page 105

Just one medium sweet potato can provide over 400% of your daily vitamin A needs!

DIRECTIONS

1. Preheat oven to 350°F. Place sweet potato tots on baking sheet in a single layer and bake for about 7 minutes.
2. After 7 minutes, flip tots over and crumble the veggie chorizo sausage over the tots. Continue baking for another 7-8 minutes.
3. Remove from oven and sprinkle evenly with vegan cheese. Return to oven and continue baking until cheese is melted (or until hot, if using Nacho Cheeze sauce), about 4-5 minutes.
4. Serve with a side of lightly steamed broccoli seasoned with sea salt.

SERVINGS	TIME	LEVEL	KCAL	FIBER	CARB	FAT	PROTEIN
5-6	25 mins	easy	392	5g	60g	14g	8g

Marcus' Sweet Heat Loaded Nachos

My brother, Marcus, is big on personality and flavor and it shows through in his cooking. This recipe is loaded with flavor, combining sweet flavors from the BBQ sauce, with a little heat from the salsa and green chilies. Marcus has fully leaned into vegan cooking and whipped up this delicious dish for him and his daughter, Mya. She gave it two thumbs up!

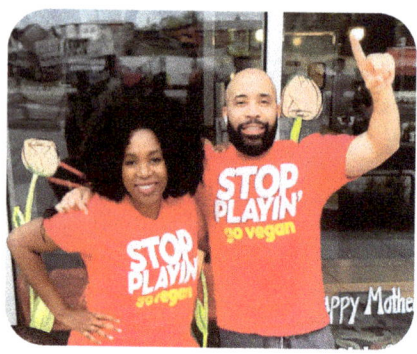

Choosing organic BBQ sauce helps you avoid additives like high fructose corn syrup, which is linked to metabolic issues & chronic disease.

INGREDIENTS

12 oz	organic lime tortilla chips
10 oz	vegan beef crumbles (i.e., Beyond Beef Crumbles or maple flavored tempeh)
½ cup	organic barbeque sauce (medium heat)
2 cups	vegan cheddar or pepper jack cheese shreds or use Nacho Cheeze recipe on page 105
15 oz	organic refried beans (1 can)
¾ cup	Hatch green chilies, diced
½ cup	coconut sour cream, page 104
½ cup	salsa, medium heat
½ cup	black olives, sliced

DIRECTIONS

1. Add vegan crumbles and BBQ sauce to medium pan and heat through, about 5-6 minutes. Set aside.
2. In a separate pan, heat refried beans with a small amount of water. Bean mixture should be loose. Stir in 1 teaspoon of chili powder and 1 teaspoon of paprika.
3. Spread tortilla chips out on oven safe platter or baking sheet.
4. Carefully sprinkle crumbles evenly on top of tortilla chips.
5. Gently spread refried beans over vegan crumbles with a spoon.
6. Sprinkle vegan cheese evenly over beans.
7. Put layered nachos in over and broil on low to medium until cheese melts, about 3 minutes. Watch closely to avoid burning chips.
8. Remove from oven and top with black olives, salsa, green chilies and vegan sour cream. Serve immediately with a side of guacamole.

SERVINGS	TIME	LEVEL	KCAL	FIBER	CARB	FAT	PROTEIN
5-6	25 mins	easy	569	9g	81g	11g	26g

Michael's Meatless BBQ Meatballs

A family favorite! My mother started with a vegetarian, fried version. Me and my brother, Michael, took the recipe and did a healthier vegan spin, removing eggs and cow's cheese and baking instead of frying. Now Michael is the meatball master!

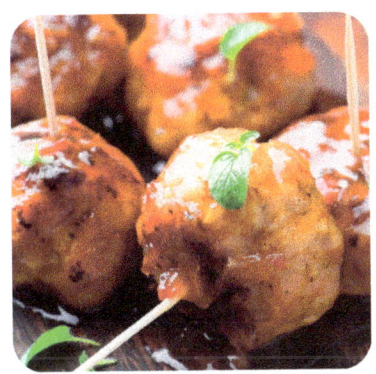

INGREDIENTS

1 cup	pecan meal
1 cup	gluten-free Italian bread crumbs
1 cup	vegan cheddar or pepper jack shreds
1 large	green pepper, finely chopped
1 large	onion, finely chopped
¼ cup	extra virgin olive oil
1 tsp	sage
1 tsp	garlic powder
½ tsp	cayenne

BBQ SAUCE:

16 oz	medium to spicy organic BBQ sauce
8 oz	organic peach preserves or orange marmalade

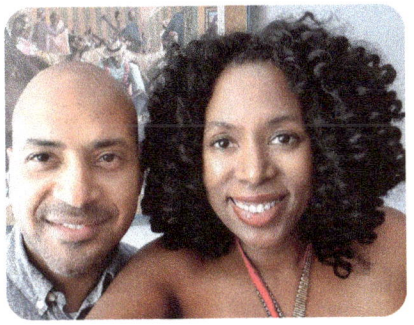

DIRECTIONS

1. Preheat the oven 375°F. Spray a cookie sheet with non-aerosol olive oil cooking spray or oil sheet with olive oil. Oil a glass baking dish (11 x 7 in.) with olive oil.
2. Mix all ingredients together in a large bowl except the sauce ingredients.
3. Mix well until all ingredients are moist and blended well.
4. Roll into small balls (about 3/4 inch diameter) and place onto the cookie sheet, evenly spaced, not touching.
5. Bake for 40 minutes, until browned & crisp on the outside. Let cool for 15 minutes.
6. Place meatballs into glass baking dish (stacking is OK after they have cooled).
7. Mix the preserves or marmalade and BBQ sauce with a whisk and pour over the meatballs until all are covered.
8. Place meatballs on the middle rack of oven and bake for 35-40 minutes. Serve hot.

SERVINGS	TIME	LEVEL	KCAL	FIBER	CARB	FAT	PROTEIN
6	90 mins	Advanced	350	4g	19g	28g	9g

Aunt Ruby's Vegan Sweet Potato Pie

This is a very "loose" translation of my Aunt Ruby's delicious sweet potato pie recipe. She was an extraordinary cook and her pies and cakes were so delicious! After I became vegan, I wanted to attempt a vegan version of her recipe. She proceeded to give me instructions like "add sugar until its sweet enough", "use twice as much vanilla extract than lemon extract", then add your spices, etc. I laughed at first; but I totally understood because that's the way I cook, more on feeling and adjusting as I go. I rarely adhere to exact measurements. This recipe will get you in the ballpark, but I don't think anyone can really replicate my Aunt Ruby's recipe – you'd have to experience it to understand. Plus her secret ingredient was her love and caring for others.

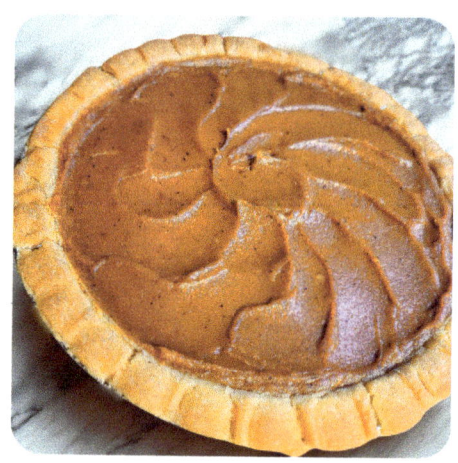

INGREDIENTS

3.5 cups	pureed sweet potatoes (about 3 large sweet potatoes, boiled, drained & peeled
1 cup	coconut sugar
¼ cup	coconut milk (regular, not light)
4 tbsp	arrow root powder
1 tsp	cinnamon
3/4 tsp	nutmeg
1/2 tsp	ground ginger
1/2 tsp	sea salt
1/8 tsp	ground cloves
1.5 tsp	organic vanilla extract
3/4 tbsp	organic lemon extract

CRUST INGREDIENTS:

1 cup	gluten free 1-to-1 baking flour
1 tbsp	coconut sugar
¼ cup	vegan butter or coconut oil (cold/solid)
6 tbsp	iced water or very cold coconut milk

A graham cracker (my favorite) or wheat pie crust can be subbed for the gluten-free pie crust.

Continued on next page.

SERVINGS	TIME	LEVEL	KCAL	FIBER	CARB	FAT	PROTEIN
8	120 mins	Advanced	359	5g	54g	15g	4g

CRUST DIRECTIONS:

1. In a bowl, whisk together the gluten-free flour & coconut sugar.
2. Add the cold vegan butter or coconut oil. Use a fork or pastry cutter to work it into the flour until the mixture resembles coarse crumbs.
3. Slowly drizzle in the iced water or cold coconut milk, mixing gently with a fork until dough just holds together when pressed. You may not need the full ¼ cup.
4. Shape the dough into a ball, flatten into a disc, and wrap it in parchment or plastic wrap. Chill for 30 minutes.
5. Roll out between two sheets of parchment paper. Transfer to your pie dish, trim edges.

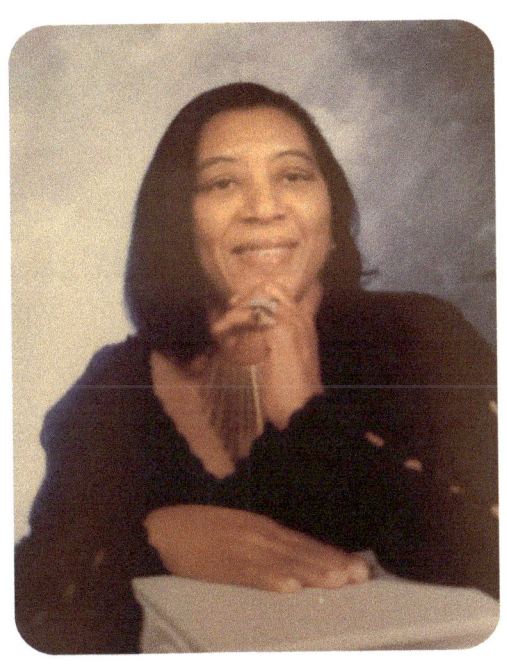

Ruby Mae Palmore Thomas

DIRECTIONS:

1. Preheat your oven to 350°F.
2. Place all pie filling ingredients into your food processor and pulse until a smooth consistency is reached.
3. Taste and adjust seasonings as desired.
4. Spoon sweet potato mixture into the pie crust and bake for 50 minutes, (edges should be set, center will jiggle slightly).
5. Remove from oven and let cool for at least 1 hour. Place in refrigerator for 3 hours or overnight to set.
6. Top with toasted coconut flakes. Slice and serve with coconut whipped cream.

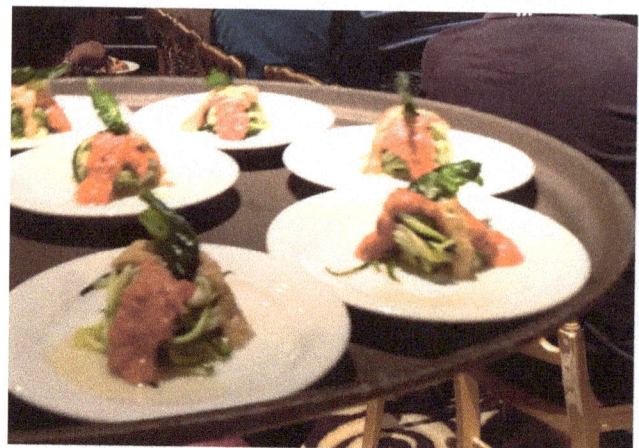

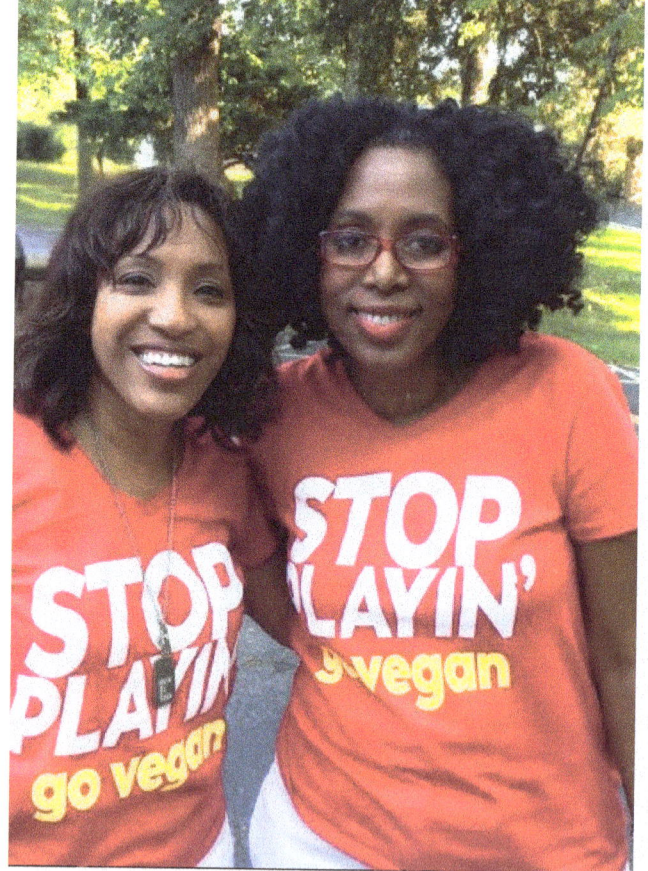

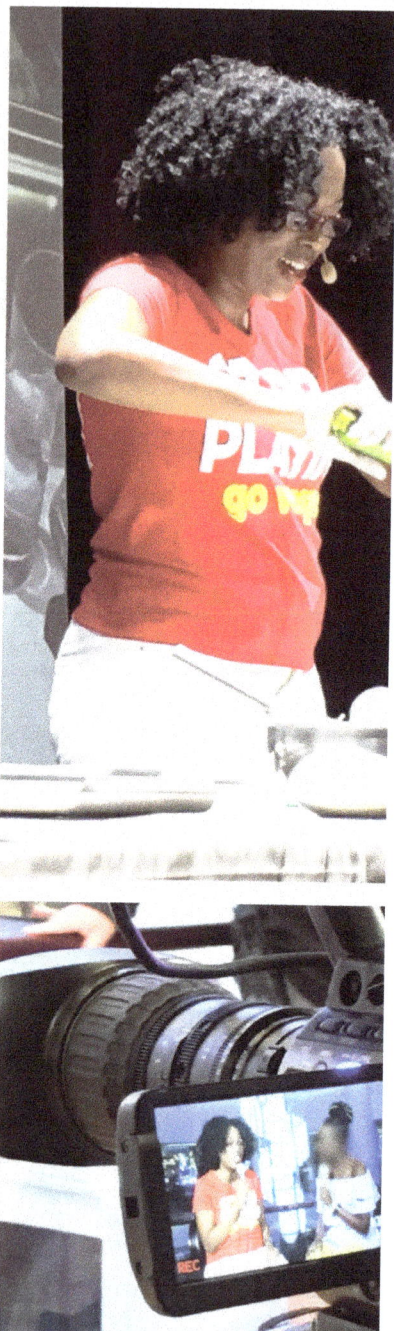

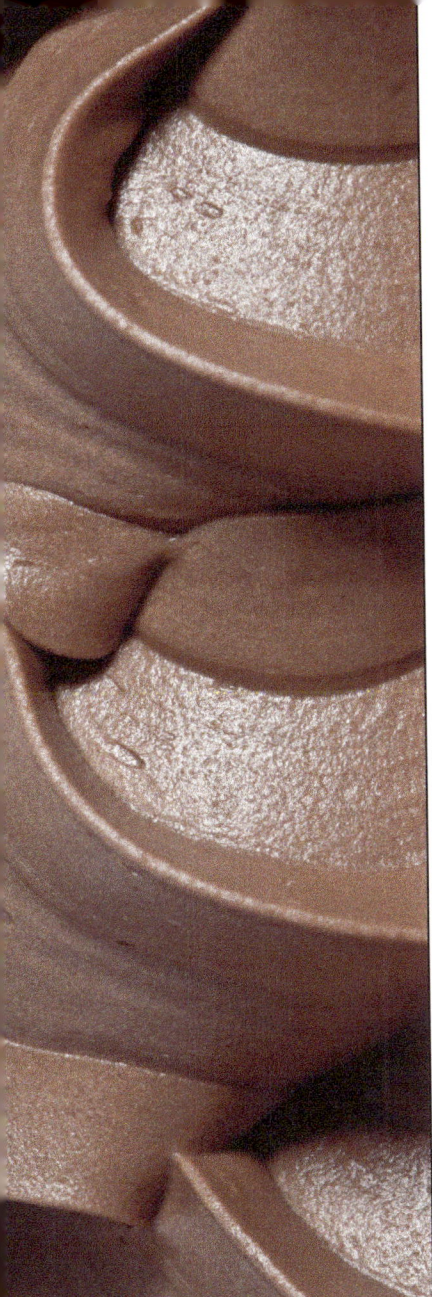

- 10 -
SWEET DECADENCE

Let indulgence feel good.

Sweet Decadence

Consider this chapter your passport to guilt-free bliss, where chocolate mousse is raw, soufflés are secretly veggie-packed, and 'ice cream' is just frozen bananas dressed up. No artificial sugars, no guilt, just ripe, vibrant flavors that happen to love you back, and won't BIG your back😄.

Each recipe here is a lesson in simplicity meeting decadence. The Chili Mango Tart? A spicy-sweet showpiece that took a few tries to perfect. The Coconut Sweet Potato Soufflé is rich, fluffy, and just happens to be made with vegetables. And the Banana Crème Pudding (my fav)? It's the hug you needed after a long day. The sweet potato cake feels like the comfort of home. And the Raw Cherry Chocolate Mousse? Smooth, rich, and irresistible. So go ahead—lick the spoon, swipe the bowl and savor the sweet decadence.

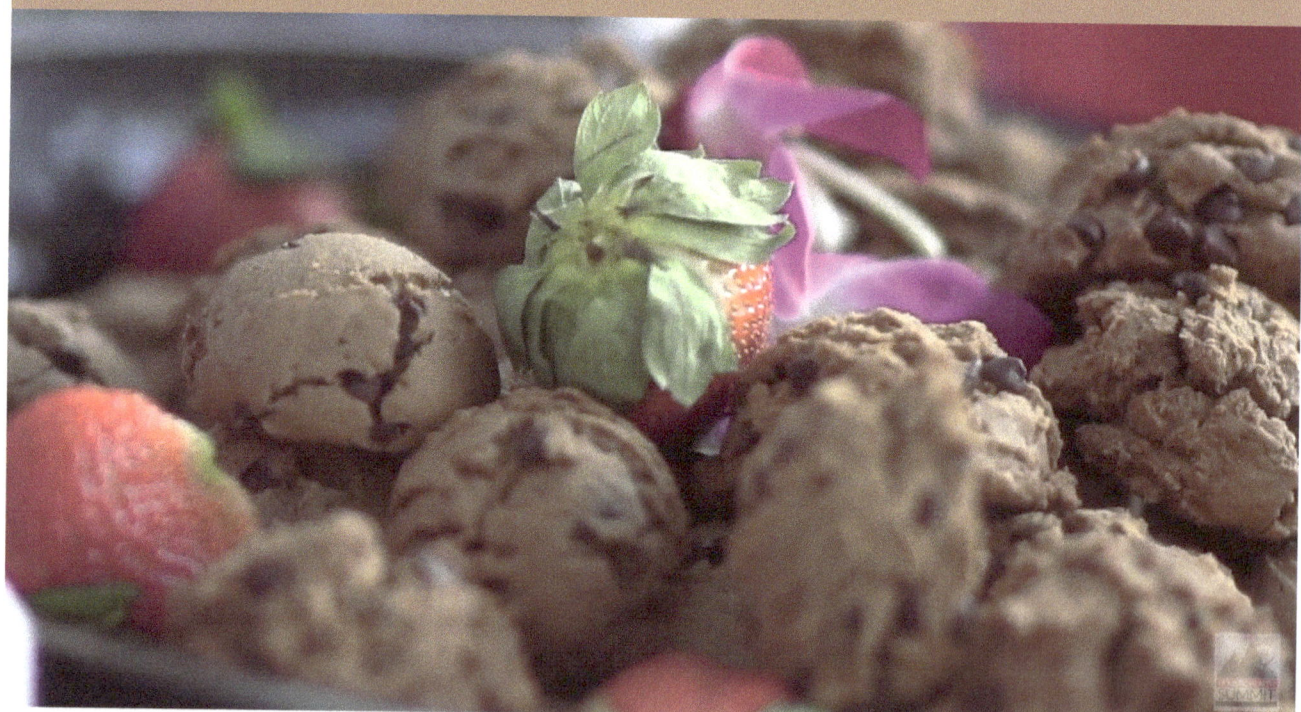

Chili Lime Mango Tart

Silky mango, sharp lime, and a slow-burn chili heat, this tart has layers!

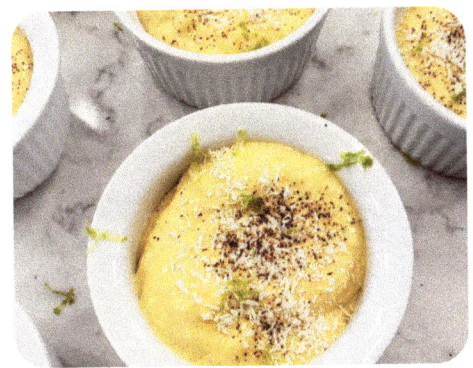

Science bonus: Chili's capsaicin clings to mango's acids, making an addictive flavor loop.

FILLING INGREDIENTS

2	mangos, peeled and chopped (2 cups)
13.5 oz	full-fat coconut milk, canned (chilled overnight or 2 hours) or 1 can coconut cream
2	limes (zest and juice of 2 limes)
¼ cup	coconut oil
¼ cup	agave nectar
½ tsp	chili powder

CRUST INGREDIENTS:

2 cups	rolled oats
1 cup	soaked pitted dates
2 tbsp	agave (optional)

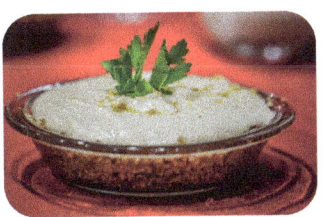

CRUST DIRECTIONS:

1. Place all the crust ingredients into a food processor and blend until it comes together into a sticky mixture.
2. Press into a 9" tart tin or into individual ramekins and refrigerate.

FILLING DIRECTIONS:

1. Chilling the coconut milk in advance is necessary to form the cream. Skim the solid part of the coconut milk (coconut cream) from the top of the can.
2. Place the mango chunks, lime juice, half the lime zest, coconut oil, agave and ¼ cup coconut cream into a food processor. Blend until smooth.
3. Pour into the large tart shell or the mini tart shells.
4. Top with remaining lime zest; sprinkle with chili powder (adjust to preference)
5. Chill in the fridge for at least 1 hour, serve cold.

SERVINGS	TIME	LEVEL	KCAL	FIBER	CARB	FAT	PROTEIN
4	60 mins	easy	495	6g	63g	28g	5g

Coconut Sweet Potato Soufflé

Some serve this as a side dish, but with its natural sweetness and fluffy texture, I say it deserves dessert status.

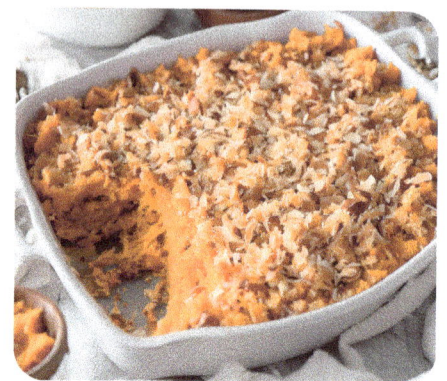

Optional: Add vegan marshmallows on top before the final bake.

INGREDIENTS

2 pounds	sweet potatoes, washed and scrubbed
1/3 cup	coconut milk
1/3 cup	raw agave nectar or dark amber maple syrup
1.5 tsp	organic vanilla extract
2 tsp	cinnamon
1 tsp	nutmeg
Dash	ground cloves
1/2 tsp	sea salt
1/3 cup	unsweetened grated coconut
1/3 cup	macadamia nuts, chopped
1 tsp	fresh lemon juice
2 tbsp	tahini (optional)

DIRECTIONS

1. Preheat your oven to 375°F. Place washed & unpeeled sweet potatoes into a glass baking dish. Bake for one hour until soft; they should be easily pierced with a fork. Remove the potatoes from the oven. Let cool for 15 minutes.
2. Peel the sweet potatoes and cut them into large pieces and place into a food processor.
3. Add coconut milk, agave, lemon juice, cinnamon, nutmeg, cloves & sea salt to food processor & pulse until smooth. Taste & adjust seasonings as desired.
4. Add grated coconut and pulse a few more times until coconut is well integrated, but not completely blended.
5. Place mixture into an oiled baking dish (9X9 inch) and smooth out with a spoon.
6. Sprinkle with coconut flakes and macadamia nuts. Drizzle with agave or maple syrup and bake at 375°F for 20 minutes; serve warm.

SERVINGS	TIME	LEVEL	KCAL	FIBER	CARB	FAT	PROTEIN
6-8	90 mins	easy	401	9g	47g	23g	6g

Sweet Potato Muffins

A cozy, naturally sweet, and spiced treat perfect for breakfast or dessert.

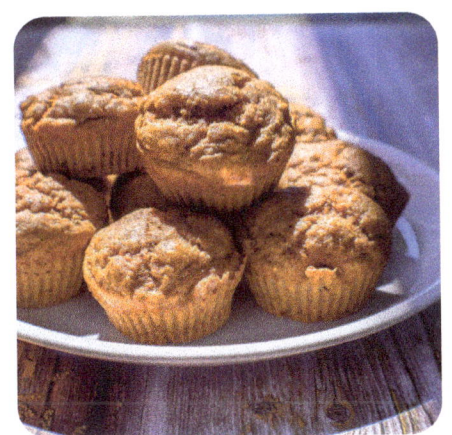

Flaxseeds replace eggs by forming a gel when mixed with water, binding the ingredients together while adding fiber and omega-3s.

DRY INGREDIENTS:

1 ¾ cups	brown rice flour or your preferred flour
1/2 cup	coconut sugar
1 tbsp	ground flax seed
1 tsp	aluminum-free baking powder
1 tsp	baking soda
1 ½ tsp	cinnamon
3/4 tsp	ground ginger
1/4 tsp	cloves
1/2 tsp	sea salt
1/2 tsp	organic raisins

WET INGREDIENTS:

1/3 cup	raw agave nectar
1/3 cup	unsweetened apple sauce
1/2 cup	coconut or almond milk
1/4 cup	water
1 tsp	vanilla extract
1 ½ cups	sweet potatoes (about 2)

DIRECTIONS

1. Preheat oven to 400°F. Spray a muffin pan with olive oil or use muffin liners.
2. Peel and shred the raw sweet potatoes.
3. Mix together all dry ingredients in a large bowl. In a small bowl, combine the liquid ingredients, except sweet potatoes. Add the liquid to the dry and mix just long enough to combine. Add the shredded raw sweet potatoes & stir to combine.
4. Spoon the batter into the muffin cups–it will be very thick. Bake for 18-22 minutes, until a toothpick comes out clean.
5. Let cool; top each of the muffins with a dollop of vanilla coconut yogurt. Makes 12 large muffins or 24 mini muffins (about 18-20 minutes).

SERVINGS	TIME	LEVEL	KCAL	FIBER	CARB	FAT	PROTEIN
12	45 *mins*	*easy*	184	2g	41g	1g	2g

Raw Cherry Chocolate Mousse

No bake decadent Chocolate-Cherry Mousse with a surprise kick of cinnamon-cayenne!
Optional whipped aquafaba adds cloud-like fluff!

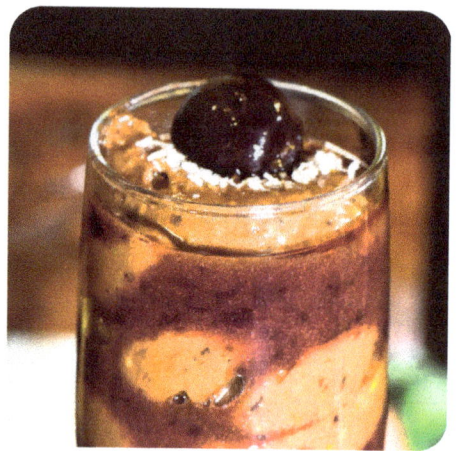

Raw cacao powder is made from unroasted beans, retaining more nutrients and bitter flavor. Cocoa powder is roasted, often sweetened & more processed.

INGREDIENTS

2 cups	pitted dark sweet cherries (frozen); reserve ½ cup cherries for garnish
2	ripe avocados
1 large	banana
1/2 cup	coconut or raw agave nectar
1/2 cup	raw cocoa powder
1 tsp	vanilla or almond extract
1 tsp	cinnamon
1 pinch	each cayenne and sea salt
1 cup	aquafaba to make more fluffy (optional)

Aquafaba is the whipped liquid from cooked chickpeas, used as an egg white substitute.

DIRECTIONS

1. Add all ingredients to food processor (except ½ cup cherries) and pulse.
2. Blend until smooth.
3. Transfer mousse to individual serving dishes or 1 large dish.
4. Chill in fridge for 2 hours. You can also freeze it to make an ice-cream like mousse.
5. Top with blended or chopped cherries and a few leaves of mint.

SERVINGS	TIME	LEVEL	KCAL	FIBER	CARB	FAT	PROTEIN
4	20 mins	easy	243	12g	38g	12g	4g

Raw Banana Crème Pudding

I love banana pudding, so here's my raw spin on the classic. Just as creamy, just as decadent.

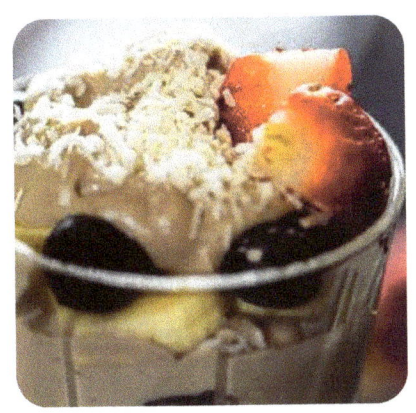

INGREDIENTS:

CRÈME:

1.5 cups	raw cashews, soak for 2 to 24 hours, drain
1/2 tsp	raw coconut or agave nectar
1/2 tsp	vanilla extract
1/8 tsp	cinnamon
2	large bananas

LAYERS:

1/2 cup	cup blueberries
2	bananas, sliced
4	strawberries, quartered
1/8 cup	shredded coconut, unsweetened

CRUST:

½ cup	raw walnuts
1	medjool date
2 tbsp	golden flax seeds, ground

Medjool dates are nicknamed 'nature's caramel', their stickiness makes them perfect for holding together no-bake crusts.

DIRECTIONS

1. Put all crust ingredients in a food processor and pulse until all ingredients are well incorporated and mixture is moist. Set crust mixture aside.
2. Put all cream ingredients into a blender and blend until mixture is smooth like cream, add a dash or two of water if needed, but not more. Mixture should be thick. It will thicken a bit more once refrigerated.
3. In 4- 6 small (6-ounce) ramekins (or use single glass dish, approximately 1 quart) scoop 1-2 tablespoons of crust mixture into ramekins and firmly press down, molding mixture into the bottom of the pan.
4. Begin layering, staring with 1 layer of cream, then sliced bananas completely cover cream, sprinkle with blueberries; repeat the layers starting with the cream.
5. Add a final dollop of cream and sprinkle with coconut; garnish with strawberries.
6. Refrigerate for at least 1 hour until completely chilled. Serve cold.

Note: cashew creme will turn a slightly tan color due to the bananas.

SERVINGS	TIME	LEVEL	KCAL	FIBER	CARB	FAT	PROTEIN
4	35 mins	intermediate	271	7g	45g	10g	4g

Banana Ice Cream - 2 Flavors

Banana ice cream mimics real dairy because freezing and blending bananas breaks down their fibers into a creamy, scoopable texture, just like churned custard.

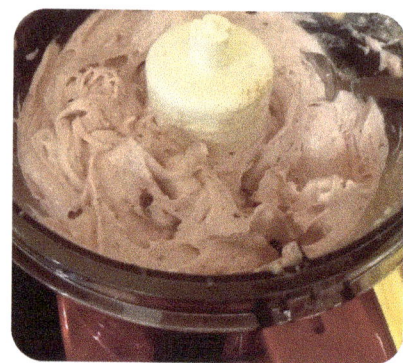

The more spotted/ripe the banana, the sweeter and richer your nice cream will taste. Flavor options are endless!

INGREDIENTS

"BUTTER PECAN" BANANA ICE CREAM

4	ripe bananas, chopped and frozen
⅓ cup	pecans
1 tbsp	maple syrup
1 tsp	vanilla extract

MANGO BANANA ICE CREAM

3-4	ripe bananas, chopped and frozen
½ cup	mango (peeled and chopped)
1 tsp	coconut nectar or agave nectar (optional)

DIRECTIONS

1. Chop bananas and let freeze overnight.
2. Remove banana from freezer and let sit for about 10 minutes
3. Put bananas and other ingredients in a food processor and pulse until ingredients are well incorporated and smooth. The mixture will become creamy, like ice cream. Do not over-process or the mixture will thaw and become runny.
4. For the "butter pecan", add all of the ingredients except the pecans, blend the bananas and then add the pecan and pulse 1 or 2 more times.

Best served immediately. *Note: Banana ice cream freezes hard; if your freeze it, let it thaw for 10 - 15 minutes before serving.*

SERVINGS	TIME	LEVEL	KCAL	FIBER	CARB	FAT	PROTEIN
4	20 mins	easy	183	4g	32g	7g	2g

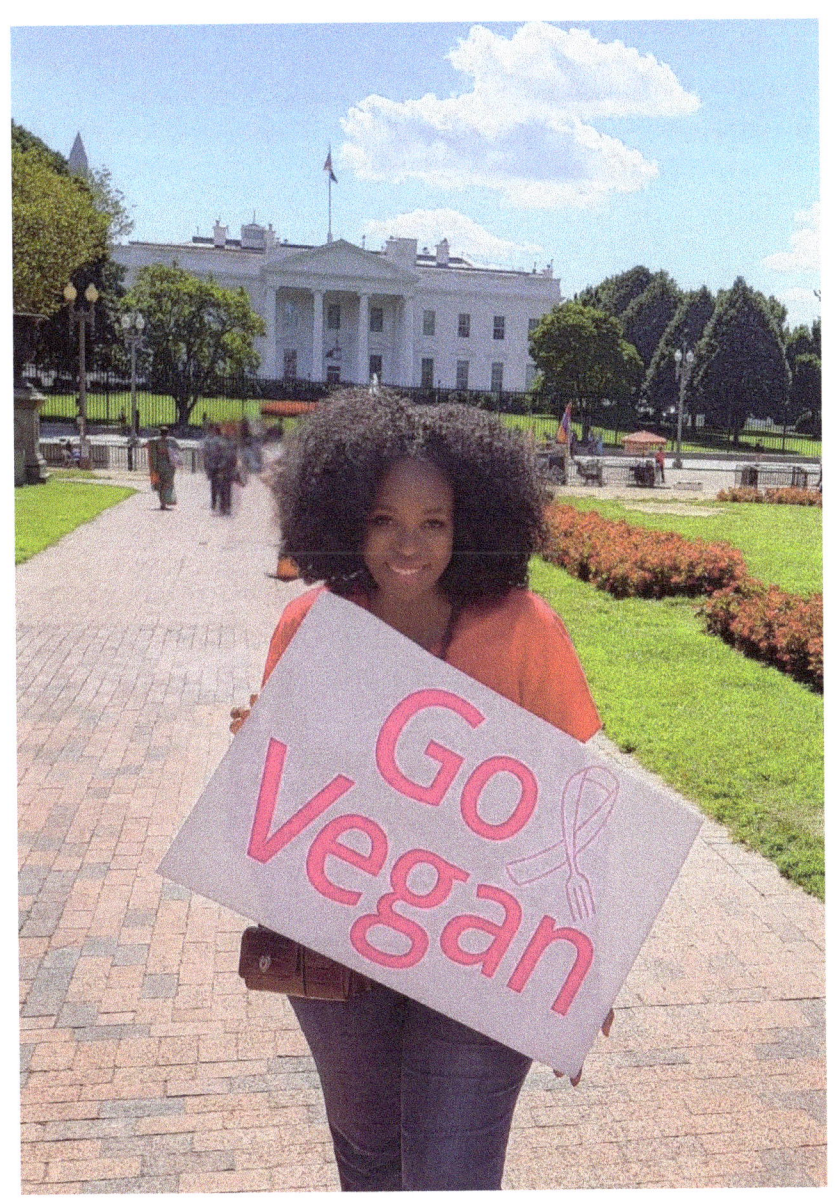

Recipes shared, taste buds sparked,
now go forth and eat plants! 🌱

ABOUT THE AUTHOR

Ruby Lathon, PhD

Holistic Nutritionist, Health Engineer & Plant-Powered Storyteller

Dr. Ruby Lathon is a force of nature—a certified holistic nutritionist, cancer thriver, and former award-winning engineer who now "re-engineers" health through whole-food, plant-based living. Featured in the groundbreaking documentaries What the Health and They're Trying to Kill Us, she's on a mission to prove that vibrant health begins in the kitchen.

When she's not teaching disease prevention through her nutrition coaching, online courses, or electrifying keynote speeches, she's running **Ruby Reds Vegan**, an organic meal delivery service serving Washington DC with ready-to-eat wellness. She's also the nutritionist behind Body Complete Rx (BCRX), a line of plant-based supplements sold at The Vitamin Shoppe.

The secret ingredient to her work? Food should heal like medicine but taste like celebration. That's why this cookbook is filled with recipes that nourish deeply and satisfy completely. After all, thriving isn't just about avoiding illness. It's about savoring the journey.

Connect:

For speaking inquiries and book signings: info@RubyLathon.com
RubyLathon.com | RubyRedsVegan.com

Index